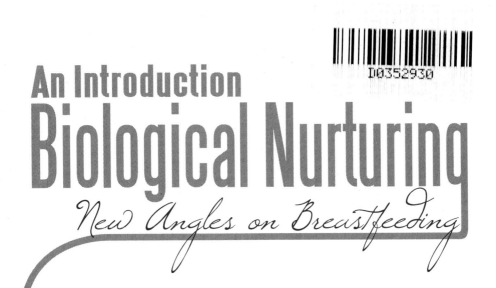

An Introduction
Biological Nurturing
New Angles on Breastfeeding

WITHDRAWN

Suzanne Colson, RM, Ph.D.

© Copyright 2010

An Introduction to Biological Nurturing
New Angles on Breastfeeding

Praeclarus Press, LLC

2504 Sweetgum Lane

Amarillo, Texas 79124 USA

806-367-9950

www.PraeclarusPress.com

DISCLAIMER

The information contained in this publication is advisory only and is not intended to replace sound clinical judgment or individualized patient care. The author disclaims all warranties, whether expressed or implied, including any warranty as the quality, accuracy, safety, or suitability of this information for any particular purpose.

ISBN: 978-1-939807-55-7

Dedication

This book is dedicated to the mothers and babies who participated in the study and to all those parents who have sent me their lovely photos. Thank you for sharing your biological nurturing experiences and giving me permission to use your pictures.

To my grandchildren, Mustafa Benjamin and Ayla Dufur, and their wonderful mother.

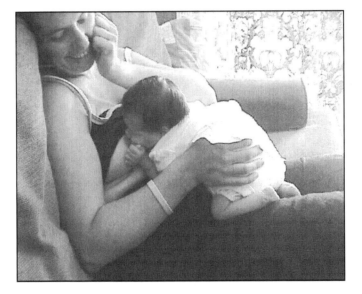

Preface and Acknowledgements

This book introduces a new approach to breastfeeding called Biological Nurturing (BN). BN is a collective term for optimal breastfeeding states and positions whose interactions release spontaneous behaviours that help mothers and babies get started with feeding. Many people are both intrigued and confused about BN, so the aim of this book is first and foremost to clarify what it is, why we need it, and the reasons for introducing new, and some would say awkward, vocabulary for an age-old art. Biological nurturing is not really 'new', but the laid-back maternal postures central to the concept are rarely portrayed in the mainstream literature, except to illustrate *incorrect* maternal posture, *important things to avoid*, or occasionally as some novel positions to try when there are problems.

Chapter 1 introduces biological nurturing as a mother-centred approach, where comfort is the priority. The BN maternal postures open the mother's body, increasing the dimensions of her torso to maximise the potential to release innate mother-baby behaviours, aiding latch and sustaining milk transfer. Biological nurturing is an evidence-based approach, and its origins, background, and development through clinical practice and research are followed by a summary of the theoretical framework in Chapters 2 to 4. In Chapter 5, the mechanisms of biological nurturing are summarised and the components illustrated.

Chapters 6 to 10 comprise in-depth examination and analysis of each BN component, clarifying salient aspects of the research methods used to explain unexpected findings. Surprisingly, the positions currently used to teach or show mothers how to breastfeed often release baby reflexes as barriers to breastfeeding, and these unexpected findings mandate introducing new breastfeeding vocabulary to clarify the positional differences and the effects of gravity. These important distinctions naturally lead to a theory and discussion about species-specificity in relation to feeding positions. Throughout Chapters 6 to 10, we explore and clarify how the BN components inter-relate and interact to release spontaneous mother-baby breastfeeding behaviours.

Skin-to-skin contact is currently identified as a causative factor associated with breastfeeding duration, yet mothers and babies in pictures illustrating biological nurturing are often lightly dressed. The reasons for this and the difference between BN and skin-to-skin contact are discussed in Chapter 11. This important chapter gives us the opportunity to go straight to the heart of biological nurturing, identifying potential positional risks and enhancing understanding of the BN concept. Finally, in Chapter 12, the act of breastfeeding is described as an opportunity to lay the foundations for a lifelong relationship; the mother-baby behaviours are the means, a sensorial language of discovery.

Introducing a new approach in any discipline is a monumental task, and biological nurturing changes some things. I am so very grateful to the midwives, nurses, health visitors, and lactation consultants who have written me with insightful comments. Some of their testimonials are included throughout the book.

I owe a great debt of thanks to Kathleen Kendall-Tackett whose editorial experience and guidance transformed an academic doctoral thesis into an easy-to-read book that summarises crucial research findings, suggesting that both mothers and babies have an innate capacity to breastfeed.

An earlier version of the BN theoretical framework was published in *Midwifery Today* under the title of "Womb to World", and I am grateful to Jan Tritten who agreed to its inclusion in this book. I would also like to thank Sue Carter and Ken Tackett for many lovely line drawings that help to illustrate the BN concept.

Last, but certainly not least, I owe a great debt of gratitude to my family. My husband, Jacques, is a computer wizard and helped with pictures and figures. My sons, Bertrand, a mathematician, helped me understand the role played by gravitational forces, and Jean-Christophe, a sociologist, offered precious advice and guidance. I am particularly indebted to my daughter, Joelle. As a breastfeeding mother, she was a constant source of inspiration, often holding and breastfeeding Ayla as she read and edited each chapter of the manuscript. Joelle's critical appraisal and comments ensure that the reality of the lived experience is fully integrated. She is a constant reminder of the amazing role mothers play in the breastfeeding relationship.

Biological nurturing is quick and easy to do. The challenge lies with understanding the releasing mechanisms and their impact upon the role of the health professional supporting breastfeeding. I hope that this book will contribute to restoring confidence in nature's biological design and in mothers' innate capacity to breastfeed.

Foreword

Dr. Suzanne Colson is one of my heroes, because her thoughtful and careful research and the conclusions she has drawn from this research have finally brought common sense into the discussion of breastfeeding. What a brilliant idea she had to videotape mothers and babies who were thought to be at higher risk for failed breastfeeding, and in so doing, demonstrated how the simple act of making mothers and babies as comfortable as possible eases and facilitates the first latch.

Colson's argument that nature and nurture are both relevant to the capacity to breastfeed is lucidly developed in this book. She doesn't require us to take one side or the other in the "nature" versus "nurture" arguments that have taken place at such length in the breastfeeding literature. Instead, she suggests that both matter, as she explains how wrong-headed assumptions of the past have led to well-meaning but misguided behaviour on the part of medical professionals who have done so much to medicalize breastfeeding.

When the principles of biological nurturing are respected, instead of feeling under pressure to memorize a list of rules about how to correctly position themselves and their babies for optimum breastfeeding, mothers are allowed comfort and respect in their first interactions with their babies. Given this, they are often surprised and delighted on observing their babies' abilities to find and latch to the breast. Performance anxiety melts away and is replaced with relief and maternal pride. It is so liberating for new mothers to realize that their babies are as talented at getting to the breast as newborn hamsters. With Colson's book, hopefully, such discoveries will become less rare among women giving birth in institutional settings. Biological nurturing has been practiced at the Farm Midwifery Center since 1970.

Ina May Gaskin, CPM, PhD (Hon)

Farm Midwifery Centre

Summertown, TN, USA

By chance, one day in 2008 I clicked on a link that led me to Suzanne Colson's website, where I found and printed one of her research articles. To my astonishment, as I read it I experienced a major paradigm shift. Colson's findings rightly called into question many of the assumptions and practices that for three decades had been accepted as dogma in the field of lactation. I was so excited by what I read that I traveled from Chicago to London to hear her speak and to meet with her personally so that I could better understand her work. As I learned more, I began spreading the word in my writing and in my breastfeeding talks. Whether my audiences were in the U.S., Hong Kong, or Japan, my reports on Colson's research always elicited the most enthusiastic responses.

In this amazing book, Colson describes logically and scientifically the insights that led her to study and document the neurological reflexes and instinctive behaviors babies and mothers bring to breastfeeding and to develop the theory and practice of Biological Nurturing. Her research findings reveal that without a deeper understanding of breastfeeding dynamics, our attempts to help mothers and babies may inadvertently undermine them.

Colson's identification of 20 of the primitive neonatal reflexes babies use to get to the breast, attach, and transfer milk is an impressive leap forward in and of itself. But her remarkable genius takes our field even further. Defying expectations, when her study mothers kept their newborns in Biological Nurturing positions after birth, even late preterm babies breastfed often and well while awake and (yes!) while asleep. This work suggests new ways to use infant state to enhance early breastfeeding and overcome problems, debunking the myth that "a hungry baby will not sleep and a sleeping baby will not feed."

But there's more. Without instruction, her study mothers triggered the right feeding reflexes in their babies at the right time, challenging the idea that for mothers, breastfeeding is a learned behavior. Do mothers have instinctive breastfeeding behaviors, too? Stay tuned!

Colson's work may also change the way we think about breastfeeding promotion. Rather than trying to persuade mothers intellectually, perhaps we should focus instead on creating a private early postpartum environment that keeps them warm, comfortable, and in body contact with their babies to trigger higher oxytocic pulsatility. Colson's theory of "hormonal complexion" has the potential to be more than just another postpartum assessment tool. It may provide us with a new lens through which we can see how mothers' hormonal levels affect maternal behavior. Helping mothers achieve an ecstatic early breastfeeding experience may prove to be our most effective strategy for promoting longer breastfeeding duration.

Colson's mentor, French obstetrician Michel Odent, changed the way we think about birth. In this book, Suzanne Colson does the same for breastfeeding. Get ready to rethink—like I did—many of your most basic breastfeeding assumptions and learn some revolutionary new ways to help mothers and babies. This book will change your life!

Nancy Mohrbacher, IBCLC, FILCA

Arlington Heights, Illinois USA

June 2010

Table of Contents

Chapter 1

An Introduction to Biological Nurturing

Biological Nurturing (BN) is a mother-centred approach to breastfeeding initiation. It consists of a range of mother and baby behaviours and positions in which maternal comfort is the priority. BN aims to increase maternal enjoyment and reduce maternal fatigue. It also specifically addresses latching and other problems that can lead to unintended breastfeeding cessation occurring during the first postnatal weeks. BN can be used as a rescue strategy for the older baby (up to 8-12 postnatal weeks).

From a biological standpoint, it makes sense that both mothers and babies would have an innate capacity to feed the offspring, ensuring the survival of the species. The BN concept is, therefore, underpinned by both "nature" and "nurture".

In the breastfeeding world, the current, dominant paradigm leans more heavily towards the "nurture" end of the spectrum. This perspective has influenced breastfeeding support since Cadogan (1748) medicalised nursing practices, leading to a science of infant feeding. The opening sentence of his essay reveals the origins of a management approach that was to become the dominant mind set.

> *It is with great Pleasure I see at last the Preservation of Children become the Care of Men of Sense. In my opinion, this Business has been too long fatally left to the management of Women, who cannot be supposed to have proper Knowledge to fit them for such a Task, notwithstanding they look upon it to be their own Province* (Cadogan, 1748, p. 3).

Hardyment (1983), an English historian, calls Cadogan's essay the first of the baby-care manuals written by the *enlightened male expert*, marking the advent of a man's discourse into the baby-care arena, an area which was previously uniquely feminine.

Early in the 20th century, Sir Frederick Truby King (1924), another enlightened physician, firmly anchored the need for medical instruction and management within the mainstream breastfeeding discourse.

Just as the whole subject of Mothercraft does not come by instinct to a woman the moment she becomes a mother, but has to be studied, so does breast-feeding require thoughtful study and competent management if it is to be a success (Truby King, 1924, p. 55).

Sir Truby King expanded management techniques to include advice suggesting that too much baby-holding would spoil babies, driving them to a feckless adulthood. Although he passionately endorsed breastfeeding, he introduced the notion of the *good baby*, requiring mothers to establish *good habits* from birth, producing "a perfectly happy and beautiful Truby King baby", writes his adopted daughter in a manual called *Mothercraft* (1934, p.4).

Learning to Breastfeed: Nature or Nurture?

Is breastfeeding innate or learned? This question is at the heart of the discourse around breastfeeding management. It is also part of a larger discussion that permeates our understanding of children's development. **Nature** refers to innate characteristics or dispositions of a person. Those supporting the nature perspective of the origins of behaviour argue that a person's capacity to act in a certain way is inborn, not learned. Simply put, an innate behaviour is a reflex or an instinct; in either case, the behaviour is spontaneous, or hardwired, genetically built into the brain before birth.

In contrast, **Nurture** means nourish, develop, to bring up (or raise), and to discipline or educate (Brown, 1993). Nurturing is learned behaviour and ranges from early feeding choices to opening a bank account for your child. The advocates of the nurture determinant of behaviour consider that the baby is born like a clean slate, ready for experiences and environmental learnings to write his behavioural capacity. Variables, such as ethnicity, age, geographic situation, education, income, social class, and other socioeconomic factors, are "nurture" (i.e., environmental) influences and central to the determination of human achievement (Slater, Hocking, & Loose, 2003).

This debate has been heated in the past; yet across disciplines, researchers now agree that both nature and nurture act and interact to influence behaviours and developmental outcomes (Elman et al., 1998; Slater et al., 2003). However, today, the innate or instinctual ways of knowing are not recognised as playing an important part in how mothers develop the capacity to breastfeed. Instead, people attribute the acquisition of breastfeeding behaviours to environmental stimulation and learning. Mavis Gunther, a well-known English obstetrician and breastfeeding expert, stated categorically that mothers lack breastfeeding instincts.

There can be no doubt in the minds of those taking care of modern Western European and American women ...that instinct does not inform the mother how to feed her first baby... which is all the more remarkable since labour which is part of the same job is more effectively compulsive. ... In the animal kingdom the initiative is often taken by the neonate, who may have the mobility and the instinctive compulsion which enable it to find the nipple, and the mother's part is to be completely inert" (Gunther, 1955, p. 6864).

This paper, published in *The Lancet*, a highly respected, peer-reviewed medical journal, may be at the root of the "nurture" dominance in breastfeeding. However, it should be noted that Gunther did not base her observations on research, but rather on her clinical experience. She was influenced by such ethologists as Tinbergen (1951) and Lorenz (1952), who studied fish, insects, and birds for the most part, not mammals. Gunther (1955) sought to clarify the causes of what she considered this "maternal deficiency", theorising that in primates, including man, mimicry takes the place of instinct. She supported her argument by citing, what was at the time, recent news about a chimpanzee born in captivity who gave birth in the London Zoo and rejected the baby. If it had not been for the kindly zoo keepers who fed it, the baby chimp would have died.

Eight years after the publication of Gunther's (1955) landmark paper, Karen Pryor, an American marine biologist who wrote one of the first books about breastfeeding for mothers, recounts the incident:

> *A chimpanzee reared in the London Zoo had never seen a baby of her own species. She was so horrified at the sudden appearance of her first baby in her nice, safe and hitherto private cage that she leapt backwards with a shriek of terror and could never thereafter be persuaded to have anything to do with her offspring* (Pryor, 1963, p. 69).

Observations like these across the industrialised world led health professionals to embrace Gunther's (1955) deterministic explanation for breastfeeding failure. Human mothers, living in a bottle-feeding culture, were deprived of the visual experience of breastfeeding as children. Like animals born and raised in captivity, this deprivation during childhood resulted in maternal rejection of the offspring at birth and the inability to breastfeed. Gunther's conclusion that women need to be taught the skills of breastfeeding set the context for breastfeeding education to lean almost entirely towards the "nurture" end of spectrum.

Shifting the Paradigm: Biological Nurturing Defined

In contrast, BN brings "nature to the fore", attempting to restore balance by shifting the paradigm back to where the "nature" end of the spectrum is once again included (Colson, 2008). It never really made sense that mothers would lack breastfeeding instincts. With this in mind, the words, *biological nurturing*, in themselves suggest that we develop the capacity to breastfeed in a variety of different ways that include both learned and innate behaviours.

BN is formally defined as a collective term for a range of mother-baby positions whose interactions appear to release both mother and baby innate behaviours, aiding breastfeeding initiation (Colson, Meek, & Hawdon, 2008). What is different in BN is that mothers neither sit bolt upright nor do they lie on their sides or backs. Instead, they lean back in semi-reclined sitting postures, usually placing the baby on top of their bodies, so the entire frontal aspect of the baby's body is facing, touching, and closely applied to their body curves or to a part of the environment (Colson, 2005a; 2005b; Colson et al., 2008).

New Ways of Thinking That Aren't Really "New"

BN is easy to describe and quick to do. The concept is multifaceted, introducing new ways of thinking about breastfeeding, although it must be said that BN is not really new. Many mothers who have enjoyed breastfeeding recognise aspects of BN in what they do; health professionals also recognise assessment techniques that they are already using to support breastfeeding.

The BN concept draws upon biological theories of early behaviours and research evidence, where available. The concept also interprets and sometimes applies the anatomy and physiology of lactation in new ways. These numerous perspectives offer a strong scientific, theoretical framework underpinning BN. The concept of "biological nurturing" enables us to start again in an attempt to de-medicalise breastfeeding, identifying some unsupported assumptions passed down by those with a more medicalised approach.

What *is* new about BN is the impact of maternal positions on breastfeeding initiation. You rarely see pictures of mothers in BN positions in mainstream literature. In fact, in hospital, mothers are often told that they are not breastfeeding correctly when they lean back, as the following testimonial received from one mother suggests.

Dear Suzanne,

My son was placed to my breast shortly after the birth and fed for about 35 minutes, and it was fabulous. The midwife was very relaxed and simply placed him there and let him do his own thing, while I laid back and relaxed! I decided there and then that breastfeeding was definitely for me, but was very apprehensive as I had heard so many negative things regarding it, and I did not know anyone who had been successful for any length of time. I am certain that if my midwife had not been so natural and chilled out about this first feed, things would have been very different for me! I was moved to the postnatal ward a few hours after the birth. It was horrendous. Nurses standing guard and scrutinising every move I made breast-wise! It was here that I heard the mantra "tummy to mummy, nipple to nose" spoken aloud. I had read about it before the birth but didn't realise it was almost treated as the law! I hate those words now; I found myself repeating them in my head and didn't dare deviate. I was also told to sit bolt upright ...I was intimidated to say the least when a line up of 3 nurses stood in front of me watching me trying to force my baby to latch on. They said I couldn't go home until I could manage to feed him ok, but I so wanted to be out of there. I tried to let him find his way to the nipple and was immediately berated for it!

Now you can see why I would have appreciated simply being told that there are alternative ways to breast feed! The hospital staff was obsessed with breast feeding without seeming to offer any practical advice except for the instructions printed in the government leaflets. I have learned now that, as a mother, your instincts CAN be trusted and that your baby is well equipped to feed himself given half a chance. I just needed someone to tell me this at the time!

Thanks again [for explaining BN which] has given me so much reassurance and a lot more confidence about things. I hope I can pass this on to any new mums I come into contact with through my peer supporting role in the future.

The Need for Different Vocabulary

A question I am often asked is whether skin-on-skin contact and biological nurturing are the same. "Why call it something else"? people ask. There are many reasons to introduce new terminology and differentiate between biological nurturing and skin-to-skin contact. A central difference has to do with the level of mother's dress. BN can be done when mothers and babies are lightly dressed, rather than always requiring direct skin-to-skin contact. This is because the positional interactions through body brushing were observed to release the reflexes, not the skin-on-skin contact. These important differences will be discussed in detail in Chapter 11.

What Biological Nurturing Does for Mothers and Babies

The BN concept has its own *raison d'être*. Biological nurturing restores balance between nature and nurture, returning to mothers their innate or hardwired capacity to mix and match those learning styles that meet their needs. It is biologically economical and advantageous that in any relationship there be both innate and acquired or learned behaviours. Time and again, in both my studies and my practice, I observed untaught-yet-fixed behavioural patterns as soon as mothers laid back (Colson et al., 2008). When you do not show mothers how to breastfeed, they often demonstrate initial bewilderment followed by a spontaneous variety of behavioural responses, suggesting that breastfeeding initiation has both "discovered and instinctual" components. These observations suggest that human mothers and babies are extremely versatile and able to breastfeed in a variety of ways. There does not appear to be one way to do it. This multitude of ways in which the breastfeeding relationship can unfold is inherent in the BN concept.

The BN concept is purposefully abstract: the mother-centredness of the strategy promotes breastfeeding as a relationship aiming to increase maternal enjoyment. Apart from the laid-back postures increasing maternal comfort, there is no over-riding component within the intervention that makes it work. There is usually no teaching involved and nothing really prescriptive to say. For example, mothers do not have to undress themselves or the baby. They do not have to prepare or sit or lie in a certain way. They do not always latch the baby and they do not have to buy things.

Instead, BN is as quick and easy to do as picking up a baby. Because it is about comfort, mothers are active agents, taking responsibility to adjust their personal degree of body slope that makes the breastfeeding part work. During episodes of BN, mothers do not look like they are trying to recall instructions or worrying about breastfeeding correctly. Instead, the positional interactions (maternal posture with the baby's position) appear to release rewarding behaviours. Many mothers are surprised at the ease with which babies can latch on and feed. This often makes them smile, giggle, and laugh. This personal freedom is powerful and appears to build maternal confidence. It also underlies a BN assumption: people often continue to do the things they enjoy.

BN is not routinely "managed", although a discrete assessment is easy to do; and in the case of problems, this assessment is made explicit. Therefore, another assumption that underpins the intervention is that breastfeeding, as an activity of daily living, does not require professional help or routine management.

Finally, biological nurturing is not about what health professionals do. It is not midwife-led, mother-led, or even baby-led. Rather BN is about establishing the give and take of the nursing couple within an autonomous relationship.

Chapter 2

Biological Nurturing:
The Origins of the Construct

Biological nurturing has been developed over the past 17 years through personal and clinical experience, research, and practice-development projects. Before looking at the research that examines what makes biological nurturing work, we need to review the roots or origins of the intervention. We also need to understand how BN was first articulated in an attempt to clarify the concept further and provide some background information on how this concept evolved.

Personal and Clinical Experience

As the mother of three breastfed babies and a former La Leche League Leader, I worked as a lactation consultant for three years at Pithiviers State Hospital, a pioneering French birth centre. Highly influenced by what I learned about the connections between birth and breastfeeding during that time, I decided to become a midwife. Upon qualification, I worked for a short time as a case-load midwife, and then returned to specialise in infant feeding, supporting both breast- and bottle-feeding mothers in hospital and the community.

Although bottle-feeding mothers sometimes have problems, more breastfeeding mothers—up to 20 a day—wanted my help. I relied upon the counselling skills acquired as a LLL Leader, together with my midwifery training, to help them (Colson, 1997a). My work with mothers ranged from simple verbal encouragement to hold the baby to more complex situations requiring clinical intervention, such as where mothers had sore, bleeding nipples, mastitis, or medical conditions, like hypertension and caesarean-wound infections. I gained experience across a wide range of different clinical situations. These typically included healthy term, pre-term, or small-for-gestational-age neonates, dehydrated and/or failure-to-thrive infants requiring readmission to hospital, and previously sick babies normalising breastfeeding in preparation for hospital discharge from Special Care.

Feeding Records

Charting feeds is part of routine postnatal midwifery assessment, and standard forms are provided by most English hospitals. Although there are small variations, feeds are recorded in a column labelled Type of Feed. Other columns indicate Amount Offered; Amount Taken; Vomit; and Urine and Bowel Output.

Although the charts were used for both breast- and bottle-feeding mothers, the information focused exclusively on bottle-feeding. For example, midwives often wrote the commercial trademark of the artificial milk drink[1] offered for type of feed, and a column for vomit appeared to be included because artificially fed babies often bring up large quantities of the commercial milk drink.

Clinical experience suggested that this column was unnecessary for breastfed babies, as they rarely have milk vomits in the first postnatal days. The amount-offered and amount-taken columns seemed to undermine breastfeeding. Midwives often noted the time at the breast as an indication for the amount taken. The record of the amount ingested was considered important because it could then be compared to pre-calculated milk volumes based upon energy requirements. At the time, this was 60-100 mls/kg/day, which is an assumption driven by a bottle-feeding culture.

Breastfeeding research demonstrates that these volumes are likely too much, especially in the first 24 hours (Hartmann & Prosser, 1984; Hartmann, 1987). Furthermore, more recent research suggests that these larger quantities of artificial milk drink may have a negative impact upon the physiological processes involved in metabolic adaptation (DeRooy & Hawdon, 2002; Hawdon, Ward Platt, & Aynsley-Green, 1992). Nevertheless, these were the volume indicators commonly used to inform all assessments of neonatal well-being. The charts in themselves seemed to plant seeds of doubt, encouraging supplementation with artificial milk drink, even when breastfed babies appeared to be thriving. I was often discouraged by the amount of time wasted crossing out the chart headings and explaining breastfeeding parameters to the mothers. See Figure 1 for a typical English feed chart.

---

1   I call all commercial breastmilk substitutes "artificial milk drink" not "baby milk", as it is commonly termed in Britain. Just as a commercial orange juice that is not made with oranges must legally be called orange drink not orange juice, baby milk that is not human should be called artificial milk drink.

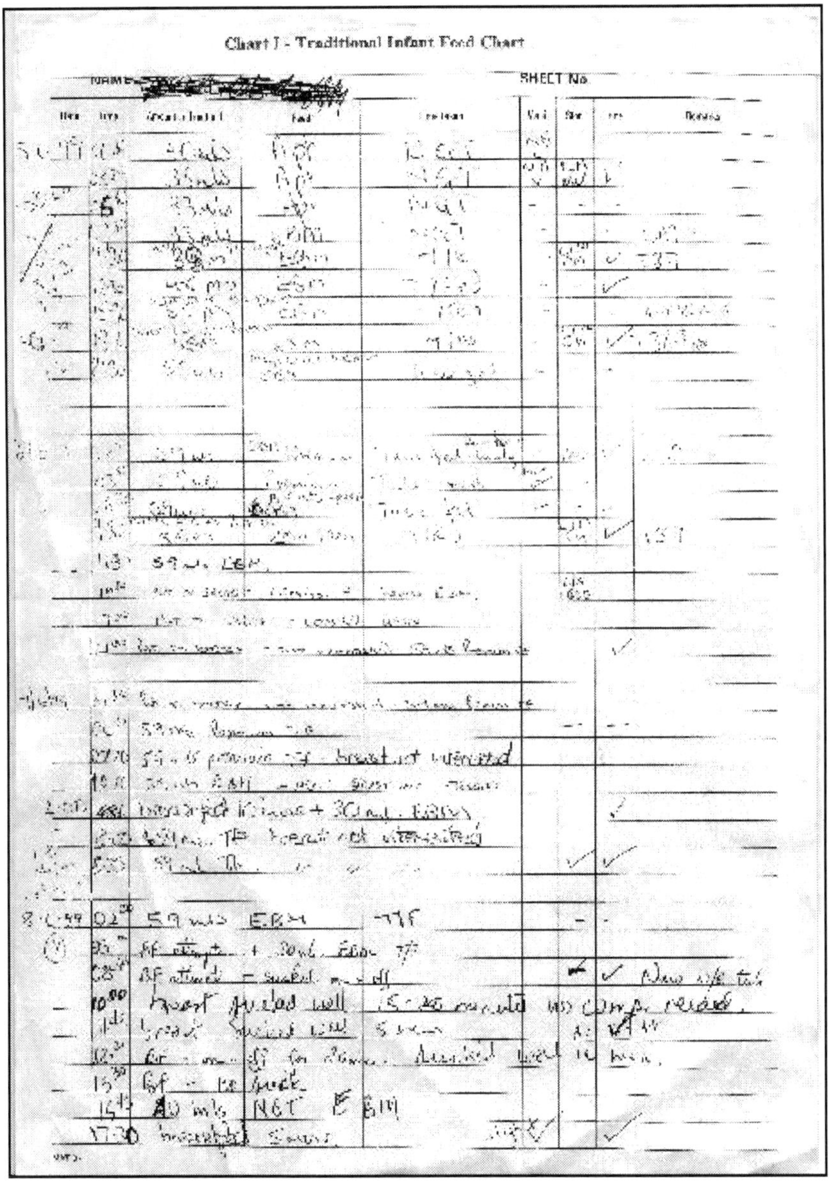

Figure 1. Typical English Feed Chart

Inspiration from a Landmark Video

Things started to change for me when I first saw Kittie Frantz's video production, *Delivery Self-Attachment*. At the time, I was a midwife/baby-feeding advisor, responsible for two busy postnatal wards in a large London hospital. This six-minute videotape (Righard & Frantz, 1992) stimulated ideas about new ways to support breastfeeding.

The video displayed clips from an observational study and showed mothers and babies in the postnatal hour following birth. The aim of the research was to examine the effects of early mother/baby separation at birth upon breastfeeding. Seventy-two mothers self-selected to one of two groups: a *contact group*, where they had at least an hour of uninterrupted skin-to-skin contact with their babies following birth or until the first breastfeed, or a *separation group*, where the neonate had skin-to-skin contact with the mother for about 20 minutes after the birth, but was then removed for measuring, bathing, and dressing before being returned to the mother.

Infants in the contact group displayed crawling, stepping, and the rooting reflex, as well as mouthing movements after about 20 minutes. At 50 minutes, most had self-attached and were sucking. Ten infants in the contact group, whose mothers received intramuscular injections of pethidine (Demerol, USA trademark), a narcotic analgesic for pain relief during labour, did not self-attach spontaneously during the first postnatal hour. Most infants in the separation group, when returned to their mothers, had no sense of direction and displayed a poor sucking technique. Righard and Alade (1990) concluded that babies should be left undisturbed in skin-to-skin contact with their mothers during the first hour following birth and that narcotic analgesia should be restricted.

These recommendations were challenged at the time, as the relatively small groups were drawn from a convenience sample, not randomised. Furthermore, the type of pain relief was not deemed relevant at the outset of the study, and therefore poorly controlled, not being held constant across the groups. Breastfeeding definitions were not made explicit, and observers of sucking technique were not blinded to the group allocation (Bragg, 1991; WHO, 1998). However, the video clips were appealing and invited discussion during my weekly antenatal education sessions for parents.

Frequent viewings prompted me to think about my practice. Further reflection led to concepts central to the development of BN as an early postnatal intervention. For example, the maternal body appeared to provide some continuity from foetus to neonate, suggesting that it would, perhaps, be an ideal nurturing environment, not only for the first hour following birth, but also during the establishment of breastfeeding. In the videotape, a clip showed the behaviour of a baby who had been separated from his mother. The baby did not appear to have a sense of direction and did not latch. However, he did make some gross rooting movements from side-to-side. I wondered whether prolonged mother-baby contact in those same close frontal positions could rescue the full reflex.

Beyond the First Hours

Mothers and babies are often separated immediately following birth for a variety of baby-centred reasons, including foetal distress, birth asphyxia, caesarean section, ventouse or forceps deliveries, prematurity, and any other intercurrent situation demanding facial oxygen or full resuscitation. Some mothers also require care necessitating separation or where baby holding is difficult. Other mothers request a meal, a bath or shower, or they feel too exhausted to hold the baby. Viewing and reviewing these video clips led to other theoretical questions:

1. Could prolonged baby holding in close body contact during the first postnatal days help to compensate for such delays in breastfeeding initiation?

2. Would it be possible for reluctant, slow feeders or those babies recovering from birth in mothers' arms to self-attach as the babies did in the video and feed well at a later stage?

The early patterns of crawling and mouthing movements looked like involuntary movement and appeared to be triggered by neonatal positions on the maternal body, even when the baby seemed to be asleep. Another question surfaced: Could all babies feed in sleep states, as the one on the video appeared to do? This got me thinking, and I made immediate changes in my clinical practice.

A Mother/Baby Suckling Diary

First, I adapted the feed charts, changing the terminology to reflect breastfeeding needs. For example, instead of being called a feed chart, it became a mother-baby suckling diary. Mothers, not midwives, kept the diary. Breastfeeding was called suckling because, by definition, suckling is a mother/baby activity, and the word in itself is abstract, playing down the need to "fill the baby up" inherent in the "feed" part of breastfeeding.

Physiological and relational grounds were introduced to encourage baby holding, using words like cues and responses borrowed from the Kangaroo Mother Care literature (Ludington-Hoe, 1993). Maternal cues were explained as those behaviours inviting the baby to feed, for example, brushing the baby's lips with the maternal nipple. Baby cues included sucking on hands or fingers, lip smacking, and rooting movements during light sleep and were discussed as early indicators of feeding readiness.

Mothers were encouraged to look for these behaviours, recording them and any other details concerning their relationship with their babies. Mothers were also encouraged to pick up their sleeping babies and hold them for long periods of time. The diaries revealed that the longer mothers held their babies, the more they fed. Therefore, the diary was expanded to include an enlarged meaning of "demand feed" to include maternal "demand." This encouraged mothers to hold and suckle their babies for as long as they wanted, regardless of the time the baby actively fed.

The routine teaching of positioning and attachment (P & A) skills during the first day quickly became unnecessary. Instead, based upon previous learnings from La Leche League, together with the growing body of evidence supporting Kangaroo Mother Care, I encouraged mothers to offer unrestricted access to the breast for as long as they wanted and as much skin-to-skin contact as they wanted. Healthy term babies are born well-fed. The key priority just after birth became "enjoyment", not feeding.

Overcoming Some Medical Hiccups

But was it safe to allow mothers to have this much freedom, without the constant charting and management by health professionals? One concern doctors immediately raised was neonatal hypoglycaemia. Hypoglycaemia, defined as low circulating blood sugar concentrations, is often seen as a risk for any baby who does not appear to be ingesting the "correct" weight/volume amounts discussed above. At the time, research by Hawdon and colleagues (1992) had been published, and their results clearly demonstrated that the healthy term breastfed neonate, unlike his bottle-fed cousin, produces ketone bodies when blood sugar concentrations are in the lower ranges of normal. It is well recognised that the human brain is an obligate consumer of glucose. Nevertheless, ketones bodies are now accepted as an alternative source of fuel for the neonatal brain during the first three postnatal days, the time of metabolic adaptation (DeRooy & Hawdon, 2002; Hawdon et al., 1992; Hoseth, Joergensen, Ebbesen, & Moeller, 2000). Called suckling ketosis, this neonatal capacity to counter-regulate is unique among mammals.

The research on suckling ketosis was not well known at the time, and the recommendations were rarely implemented in clinical practice. I raised the issue of suckling ketosis with the consultant neonatologist at the hospital, showing her some of the pilot diaries. These recorded a clear and frequent feeding trail that served to convince her that these babies were getting enough through exclusive breastfeeding. The suckling diary worked a treat with any healthy baby at risk of hypoglycaemia. See Figure 2 for the pilot suckling diary.

Mother/Baby Suckling Diary

Chart Number: 2
Days old: 2

OSA

Mothers Name	Baby's Name	DOB	Gestation	Birth Weight	Ward
		19/3/98	36/40	2160	ONS Bed 1K

Date and Time	Temp	Suckled for i.e.. breast contact	Sucked for i.e., active suckling	PU and/or BO	Supplement Not Needed / Needed & Why: Amount Given & How (cup bottle etc)	Blood Glucose (TBG)	Weight	Remarks, colour SBR, active, lethargic awake, alert, sleeping etc.
11·05 7/6·40	No T.	½ hour	½ hour			2·71	2070	sleeping baby occasional little appears... Slade super
2·45/3·50	No T.	¾ hour	short 20 mins					
6·10/6·40	warm	½ hour	No sucks					
7·odah	warm		25 mins		Strong Sucks.			Little Wee
9·5/8·00	No T.	No Sucks.			Just lying on Breast.			poo poo poo.
10/30 /10·50	warm	strong Sucks.						
1·30/1·45	No T.	15 min. Suckling			Extra Suckling.			loss of sneezing.
3·30/ 3·30	warm	strong Suckling			Extra strong Suckling	4·4·180		
4·30 - 4·45		Extra Suckling after	nappy change					poo poo poo
0·8·30·		20 warm	No wet nappy yet. strong Sucks					
11·10·12·0·		Suckled and Suckled				2060		

SBR 141
TBg 2·5

Suzanne Colson, Air call UCH 325   Breastfeeding Study   Pilot 02/98   Mother/Baby Suckling Diary

Figure 2. Pilot Suckling Diary

Clinical practice revealed that many mothers suckled their babies for long periods. They often continued at home and shared their experiences through clinics and/or letters. Community midwives and health visitors often telephoned seeking more information. They saw a difference in mothers who spent lots of time holding the baby. Suckling, as defined in the diary, appeared to increase maternal confidence and restore ownership and control. It appeared to make breastfeeding feel easier–and more instinctive.

During the three years it took to develop the diary, there were many anecdotal clinical experiences of healthy, but problem feeders or healthy at-risk babies (moderately pre-term, small-for-gestational-age infants, babies of diabetics) whose mothers were able to breastfeed exclusively using the suckling diary. Our breastfeeding rates at hospital discharge were 75% (Colson & Griffiths, 1996; Colson, 1997b). However, the reasons for this success were unclear. Whilst I thought that using the suckling diary was the single most important factor, I continued to observe a number of simple reflex-like movements that appeared to stimulate breastfeeding behaviours.

Chapter 3

How Does It Work?
The Theoretical Framework

When mothers and babies remain in close skin-to-skin and/or body contact following birth, oxytocin is released simultaneously in mother and baby. This stimulates the metabolic transition from womb to world and releases behavioural effects that promote bonding and breastfeeding (Bystrova et al., 2007; Christensson et al., 1992; Colson et al., 2008; Matthiesen, Ransjo-Arvidson, Nissen, & Uvnäs-Moberg, 2001; Nissen et al., 1996; Uvnäs-Moberg, 1996). The mammary gland is programmed to take over from the placenta. It is well-known that birth is characterised by separation, rupture, and discontinuity, yet the mammary gland offers potential for continuity during the time of postnatal transition from foetus to neonate (Colson, 2002).

Continuity and discontinuity are child-development terms referring to both the stability and change that characterise different stages of growth (Slater et al., 2003). At birth, the baby inevitably moves from the womb environment–a dark, warm, wet, sheltered place where sound is muffled and movement is restricted–to the colder, dry, bright, loud conditions of the world where there are no boundaries, and the umbilical cord is severed (Colson, 2002). The baby must adapt to life without placental support and make well-known physiological changes requiring cardiovascular, pulmonary, thermal, vestibular, immune, and metabolic adaptation.

These sudden alterations have characterised birth as one of the most dangerous times during the life span (Montagu, 1965; Thureen, Deacon, Hernandez, & Hall, 2004). However, when we look closely at foetal development, there are many points of potential neonatal continuity at birth that can help keep babies safe throughout this transition into the world. For example, there is a potential for nutritional, thermal, reflex, and continuity in behavioural state as the mammary gland takes over from the placenta. Within each one of these potential points of continuity lays special and extra maternal protection during the time of postnatal adaptation. That is, if and when mothers spontaneously hold their babies in as much skin-to-skin contact as they desire, the maternal body maintains its primary protective functions and continues to meet the needs of the new baby (Colson, 2002; Colson, DeRooy, & Hawdon, 2003).

Keeping the baby on the mother's body is keeping the baby in the right place at the right time: what Nils Bergman (2010) calls the right "habitat". It is continuity with the mother (familiar voice, heartbeat, odour, body space) that optimises the environmental conditions necessary for postnatal adaptation. That is why I often call biological nurturing a bridging strategy.

Continuity for Mothers

Giving birth is also fraught with change for the mother. During pregnancy, mothers carry their babies constantly. It would be silly to suggest that they put them down. However, as soon as the baby is born, the mother is advised to keep the baby in a cot or bassinet by her bed. Clinical and anecdotal experiences suggest that many mothers feel "empty" following birth. De Gasquet (2005), a French maternity doctor, suggests that the act of giving birth opens the maternal pelvis and mothers often experience anxiety because the womb, now being empty, needs closure. Biological nurturing, used as a bridging strategy, minimises early maternal/neonatal separation and may help with physical or psychological closure. The nurturing/nurturance role of the maternal body that so strongly underpins BN is made explicit, inviting acknowledgment of a simultaneous symbiotic/separation paradox. Mothers may wish to say they feel empty, or they might not feel so empty whilst holding the baby.

Metabolic Adaptation

Biological nurturing can also be used as a bridge to help newborns achieve metabolic adaptation. Having received a constant supply of glucose via the placenta during intrauterine life, healthy term infants are born well-fed (Colson, 2002). At birth, when the umbilical cord ceases to pulsate, this constant energy influx abruptly stops. The neonate must adapt to the feasting/fasting patterns of extrauterine life, maintaining normal blood glucose concentrations (DeRooy & Hawdon, 2002; Hawdon, Ward Platt, & Aynsley-Green, 1992). Research evidence indicates an association between longer inter-feed intervals and lower blood glucose concentrations, putting some babies at risk of neonatal hypoglycaemia (Hawdon et al., 1992; Hoseth et al., 2000; DeRooy & Hawdon, 2002).

BN often increases feeding frequency, thus reducing the interval between feeds (Colson, 2000; Colson et al., 2003). For example, during metabolic research projects carried out in London hospitals, one participating mother of a healthy, but moderately preterm baby born at 34 gestational weeks held her baby for 16 of the first 24 hours (Colson et al., 2003). That preterm baby, who would have normally been transferred to special care and tube-fed for the first postnatal hours/days, maintained blood glucose concentrations within normal limits throughout and was exclusively breastfed from birth. Taken together, the above evidence, ranging from trials to a case study, suggests that mothers should be encouraged to use biological nurturing for at least the first three postnatal days, the time of metabolic adaptation.

Continuity in Maternal Oxytocin

Biological nurturing may also provide more continuity for mothers, specifically in regard to their oxytocin levels. Oxytocin is released both centrally and peripherally before and after birth, with maternal blood concentrations rising during the third trimester of pregnancy (McNabb, 1997a; Uvnäs-Moberg, 2003). Oxytocin must be released in a pulsatile fashion to be effective. Nissen and her colleagues (1996) have shown that oxytocin pulsatility is higher in the first hour following birth than at any other time.

Oxytocin is known as the contraction-and-ejection hormone. High maternal concentrations may, first and foremost, be a protective mechanism, maintaining the uterus well contracted, thus decreasing the risk of primary (first 24 hours after birth) postpartum haemorrhage (Bullough, Msuku, & Karonde, 1989). High oxytocin pulsatility on the second postnatal day has also been associated with longer breastfeeding duration (Nissen et al., 1996). Taken together, this research evidence suggests that encouraging close body contact between mother and baby for the first six weeks may increase and prolong high oxytocin pulsatility, supporting breastfeeding duration, as well as offering further protection against secondary (the first six postnatal weeks) postpartum haemorrhage. Six weeks is also the time that corresponds to the establishment of breastfeeding.

Early Breastfeeding and Mother's Milk Supply

Early breastfeeding patterns frequently differ from those established later, both in type, frequency, and duration, often changing on a daily basis. For example, there is no uniformity in the first 24 hours. Babies left in cots may not feed at all for eight hours or longer. During BN, babies may latch on and suck often, but the length of each episode may be very short. The first-day patterns are often followed by periods of constant suckling during the second and third postnatal days, suggesting that arbitrary time schedules are inappropriate (Howie et al., 1981). This feeding frenzy coincides with the time when many mothers fear they have not got enough milk. Biologically, this fear appears to be unsubstantiated, as research findings suggest that the mechanisms for mother's breast-milk production are fully developed at about four gestational months (Hytten, 1995), with many mothers releasing small quantities of milk during pregnancy (Brown & Hurlock, 1975).

Mothers who miscarry often, regrettably, have copious milk production (Reader, 1996). However, high concentrations of oestrogen and other pregnancy-maintaining hormones inhibit milk release (Hytten, 1995). The fear that many mothers experience concerning milk insufficiency can be aggravated by well-intentioned, but erroneous information they receive about how their milk will "come in" on the third postnatal day. Physiologically, this appears to be incorrect as the milk arrived during pregnancy (Colson, 2007; Hytten, 1995). On or around the third postnatal day, it is only the milk volume that increases to meet the baby's increasing needs. Initially, babies only require small, frequent amounts of colostrum, which is the first milk (Hartmann & Prosser, 1984; Hartmann, 1987). It is an advantage that there is not a copious milk supply in the first days, as these frequent but short feeds help the baby organise sucking and swallowing with breathing.

We have known for many years that suckling is an important factor associated with milk production, promoting high concentrations of prolactin, the milk-producing hormone (McNeilly, Robinson, Houston, & Howie, 1983). In contrast, the release of oxytocin can be stimulated by merely thinking about the baby, with a mean peak in pulsatility at two and one-half minutes. Except in the period immediately following birth, prolactin is only stimulated through mother/baby suckling, that is, face-and-hand-to-breast contact and active milk extraction, with prolactin pulsatility peaking at 35-40 minutes from the start of a breastfeed (Howie, 1985; Uvnäs-Moberg, 2003).

These research findings indicate that initially it is lots of baby holding and breast emptying that regulates maternal milk supply, and we need to make that explicit to mothers. When starting out with breastfeeding, one feed often blends into the next. Many mothers say that they cannot put their baby down. We need to tell mothers that this is normal. Mothers often think that because the baby cries when they put him down, they have not got enough milk. That is usually a misinterpretation. The baby cries when they put him down because he is no longer in the right place. The biological argument suggests that during at least the first three postnatal days–the time of metabolic adaptation–it is not normal to put the baby down for long periods of time.

The Contrast: Modern Lactation Management

In contrast to BN, there is the current framework of lactation management. During the 1980s, following the publication of the landmark studies examining the anatomy of infant suckling, lactation management was considered essential to achieve successful breastfeeding, and step-by-step management components were developed simultaneously across the English-speaking world (Woolridge, 1986a; 1986b). Although Woolridge and his colleagues only studied the events happening in the neonate's buccal cavity, clinical applications of their research findings standardised the maternal positions, skills, and techniques taught to mothers (Woolridge, 1986a; 1986b).

Like the active management of labour, fixed systems of lactation management were created to show mothers how to breastfeed. Midwives were told first to advise mothers how to position themselves with an upright back at right angles to their lap or lying on their sides. Then mothers were taught how to hold the baby in one of three ways: the cradle, cross cradle, or the clutch or rugby/football hold, sometimes placing him on a pillow, sometimes on their laps, and to attach the baby to the breast correctly, bringing baby to breast with nipple to nose, and leading in with the chin following mouth gape (see Figure 3).

In that way, the proponents of breastfeeding management suggested that a close "asymmetrical" latch is achieved, where more of the lower part of the maternal areola is in the baby's mouth.

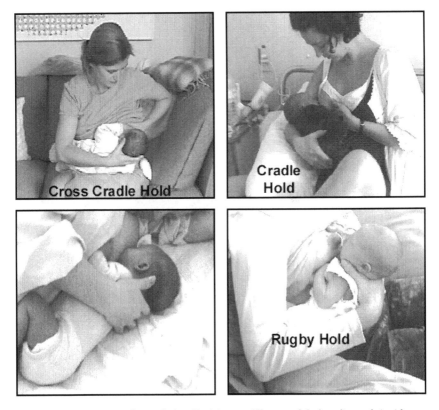

Figure 3. Mainstream Breastfeeding Positions and Postures Mothers lie on their sides or sit upright using three standardised baby holds. Photos © Suzanne Colson.

When I undertook an extensive literature search for my PhD, I could not locate any research data to support these postural/positional recommendations. However, I did find some interesting grey literature. In her PhD research, Sulcova (1997), a behavioural psychologist, reports maternal feeding observations in descriptions of spontaneous mother/baby behaviours. This mother/baby choreography underpinned the Prague Newborn Behaviour Description Technique, an assessment instrument providing information on the healthy newborn's level of well-being through observations of maternal/infant behavioural interactions. As a component, Sulcova observed the breastfeeding techniques of mothers who were taught positioning and attachment skills, either sitting upright or side-lying. Sulcova (1997) describes tension laden and unbalanced maternal sitting postures, suggesting that mothers will always sacrifice their personal and positional comfort for a good latch.

Biological Nurturing: Keeping Mothers and Babies Together

In practical as well as biological terms, the nutritional, developmental, and emotional needs of the newborn infant are met through suckling in close body contact (McNabb & Colson, 2000; Christensson, Cabrera, Christensson, Uvnäs-Moberg, & Winberg, 1995). In a protected and unhurried environment, physiological beacons of smell may light the way to the breast (Righard, 1995; Varendi, Porter, & Winberg, 1994). During the first days of extrauterine life, the newborn demonstrates instinctive actions for finding and latching onto the breast (Colson et al., 2008; Odent, 1977; Pryor, 1963; Widstrom, Ransjo-Arvidson, Matthiesen, Winberg, & Uvnäs-Moberg, 1987; Winberg, 1995).

Mothers also demonstrate natural preferences for baby holding, and during episodes of BN, they were observed to place their babies up their bodies to help them find the breast (Colson et al., 2008; De Château, 1987). Even though certain labour-ward practices may mask this instinctive competence (Righard & Alade, 1990), biologically it appears to be the close ventral juxtapositioning between mother and baby that elicits reciprocal mother-baby inborn breastfeeding behaviours.

The full contact between the baby's body on top of the mother's body seems to release baby reflexes, while the sight and smell of the baby, together with his movements and sweet noises, seem to elicit spontaneous maternal responses (Colson, 2002). In a relationship, there is not one person who always leads. Rather it appears to be a chicken-and-egg phenomenon, where it is impossible to say which one is the initiator. Like in so many relationships, "who initiates" quickly becomes irrelevant.

As early as 1954, Grantly Dick-Read, pioneering obstetrician for "childbirth without fear", summarised maternal biological capacity. He claimed that breastfeeding satisfies all the baby's needs for warmth, security, and food. These claims have always made common sense. Research findings now support common sense. Building upon a potential for continuity in the transition from foetus to neonate, biological nurturing is a back-to-the-future strategy that builds upon Grantly Dick-Read's work. Is it not time to talk about "breastfeeding without fear"?

In summary, taken together with some early research evidence from the 1970s and 1980s demonstrating neonatal competence (Brazelton, 1973; Leboyer, 1974; Klaus & Kennel, 1976; Klaus & Klaus, 1985), the effectiveness of Kangaroo Mothering Care (Ludington-Hoe, 1993; Anderson, Moore, Hepworth, & Bergman, 2003), and the physiology of metabolic transition (Hawdon et al., 1992), it is clear that breastfeeding is a complex biological and nurturing relationship. The next step for me was to understand the role of BN in this process and that required research.

Chapter 4

Exploratory and Descriptive Research: The Background Studies of Biological Nurturing

In 1997, Jane Hawdon, the pioneering metabolic researcher whose work influenced my practice, advertised for a research midwife. In a bi-centre randomised controlled trial, Hawdon and Williams, another leading consultant neonatologist, were examining the effects of supplementation upon breastfeeding and metabolic adaptation for healthy, but moderately pre-term infants. Hawdon and DeRooy, one of her senior medical registrars, were also carrying out similar metabolic profiles for healthy, but small- and large-for-gestational-age term babies. Supplementation was, prior to this research, routinely prescribed for these healthy, but vulnerable babies considered at risk of hypoglycaemia. I jumped at the opportunity to work under their guidance and was seconded to the new position.

Having had clinical, albeit anecdotal, experiences of supporting exclusive breastfeeding for mothers whose babies were vulnerable, but otherwise healthy, it was exciting to have close clinical supervision from experts like Hawdon, DeRooy, and Meek, another senior medical registrar. Their supervision sharpened and enhanced my clinical assessment skills. The concepts of suckling ketosis and counter-regulation came to life.

An Exploratory Pilot Study

A feeding diary had originally been part of the research protocols, but had been abandoned because no one could be bothered to complete it. Everyone just used the feed charts. Hawdon agreed that the mother/baby-suckling diary could be used in addition to the feed charts. During the nine months of the secondment, I recruited over 50 mothers to the metabolic trial and piloted the suckling diary with 12 of them to explore biological nurturing (termed biological suckling at the time) as a strategy for a subset of mothers recruited for the metabolic studies who wanted to breastfeed exclusively.

Using a qualitative methodological approach, the aims were first to articulate biological nurturing as an intervention and second to examine if, and how, BN affected breastfeeding initiation. The suckling diary was the main data collection instrument. The metabolic research protocols were flexible, and when babies were breathing air, appeared healthy, and were infection free, the research midwife supervised their care on the postnatal ward.

I studied 11 healthy, but moderately preterm babies (between 34 and 36 weeks gestation), and one healthy, but small-for-gestational-age baby; all were breastfed from birth. A key finding was that many healthy, but moderately pre-term infants can breastfeed exclusively from birth. Clinical midwifery and breastfeeding assessment skills, reflecting an understanding of metabolic adaptation, were crucial to avoid unnecessary supplementation. Full results of the pilot study, undertaken for a MSc in midwifery,[2] are published elsewhere (Colson, DeRooy, & Hawdon, 2003). However, reviewing certain temporal findings, or spontaneous mother-specific breastfeeding styles, can help clarify the background concepts behind biological nurturing.

Temporal Findings

Biological nurturing measures temporal variables of two behavioural types: body/breast contact and active sucking. Through analysis of the diaries, I was able to calculate simple statistics for such proximate variables as suckling frequency, duration, and interval duration defined by Quandt (1998) as key biological factors that impacted breastfeeding initiation. For example, for three of the mothers who spontaneously held their babies at birth, the mean holding time was one hour, ranging from 45 to 90 minutes. This replicated other findings (De Château & Wiberg, 1977; Righard & Alade, 1990), adding to an increasing body of evidence, suggesting that the first hour following birth offered a critical or sensitive window of time. Interestingly, mothers did not record if they held their babies in skin-to-skin contact. At the time of this study (1998), it was not yet standard practice for all mothers to hold their babies in skin-to-skin contact.

The First 24 Hours

One of the first variables I examined was the number of BN episodes that occurred in the first 24 hours. An example of what we coded as a BN episode included the time the mother spent holding the baby in positions where the baby had unrestricted access to the breast in as much skin-to-skin contact as desired versus the time the baby actually spent actively feeding.

---

2 The MSc dissertation was awarded distinction in June, 2000, and a bound copy is available for consultation at London South Bank University Library

Active feeding was defined as sucking bursts with visible and/or age specific audible swallowing.

The number of BN episodes varied quite a bit, ranging from 7 to 18, with a mean of 12. The neonates had unrestricted breast contact for a mean total of 7 hours and 40 minutes. However, there was a broad range in the breast contact time, with three mothers holding their babies in unrestricted breast access for approximately 4 hours and one mother for 16 hours. During the first 24 hours, babies actively breastfed, with vigorous sucking action, for a mean total of 2 hours and 35 minutes.

Those contact and active feeding times were longer than the time parameters in the new hypoglycaemia feeding guidelines that the midwives used on the ward (National Childbirth Trust, 1997). In the guidelines, mothers were not encouraged to hold their babies outside of active feeding; the midwives, therefore, advised mothers to gently arouse sleeping babies after eight or 12 postnatal hours if they had not yet awakened for a feed.

Mothers often ask questions about the length of time they should hold or feed their babies. The range of those findings was so wide, corresponding to individual needs, that it was difficult to give any fixed guidance. This is the reason why uniform temporal suggestions are absent from the "how to do it part" of biological nurturing. The above findings, with the wide range of times, suggest that we should not give mothers specific numbers about how long they should hold or feed their babies. Just as the definition of neonatal hypoglycaemia is not a numbers game (DeRooy & Hawdon, 2002), frequency of body contact and active milk transfer cannot be numbered, although sometimes it is helpful to give a time range. Suggesting, for example, that mothers hold their babies a lot, maybe a third of the day, works well for many.

One way to respond to mothers' temporal questions is to ask how long they *want* to hold the baby, and then agree with her response if it is within those research parameters. Tell her that the evidence suggests that the number she gives is spot-on accurate. Another way to respond to mothers' questions about how long they should hold their babies during the first 24 hours is to remind them that this time yesterday they were feeding the baby constantly and they could not put him down. This often makes mothers laugh. Laughter is such an important part of parenting, often clarifying the common-sense responses.

Attending midwives and doctors also need indications of normal parameters to inform assessments. Without generalising, these statistics did just that, helping to frame temporal and frequency issues in a non-prescriptive way.

At the time, I was unaware of the central role played by the mother's posture. Nevertheless, during episodes of BN, I observed and described 10 primitive neonatal reflex-like movements that appeared to stimulate feeding behaviours for the healthy, but vulnerable babies studied. The presence or absence of the baby reflexes helped to determine clinical management, as well as breastfeeding support.

Even if a baby-reflex movement was only weakly present, I found it could release a cascade of innate baby behaviours. Seven of the twelve at-risk babies that I studied required no supplementation with artificial milk drink from birth. The mean age at hospital discharge was six days, and all 12 infants were exclusively breastfed at that time. At four postnatal months, 11 of the 12 infants were still breastfed (10 exclusively). Study numbers were too small to enable comparisons. However, these results looked encouraging when viewed alongside the UK national statistics. My findings on exclusive breastfeeding were unusual at the time for any healthy baby, let alone healthy, but moderately preterm or small-for-gestational-age babies.

Although the diary was particularly helpful for first-time mothers, others found it a bit of a chore, and only completed it because it was part of the research protocol. At the same time, I was developing an increased awareness of the role of the reflexes. I, therefore, attributed the achievement of these high rates of exclusive breastfeeding to the systematic release of the baby reflexes in BN positions, not the diary. The increase in breastfeeding duration across the small number of mother-baby pairs studied suggested that further research looking at biological nurturing was warranted (Colson, 2000; Colson et al., 2003).

The PhD Study of Biological Nurturing

These previous studies highlighted that keeping mothers' and babies' bodies together had a positive impact on breastfeeding. It was this observation that led me to investigate what I now describe as biological nurturing. During the background studies, the how-to's of BN were more or less defined, identifying what looked like ten primitive neonatal reflexes stimulating breastfeeding. However, if BN was to become a valid and reliable breastfeeding intervention, we needed further research to clarify the concepts and understand the underlying mechanisms.

Selecting a Research Design

All the mothers in the pilot study of BN were breastfeeding at six weeks. It was therefore tempting to pilot a randomised controlled trial (RCT), hypothesising that biological nurturing releases primitive neonatal reflexes and increases breastfeeding duration. A trial would allow me to compare two groups: BN as the experimental group, and a positioning-and-attachment-skills-teaching group as the control. However, a hypothesis implies that the theory supporting the intervention is well developed and that the components are fully identified and defined operationally (Medical Research Council, 2000). Following the pilot study, neither of these criteria was fully met.

As discussed in the previous chapter, the concept of biological nurturing was purposefully abstract. A literature search revealed that many researchers have studied rooting and sucking, but few have looked at the role other PNRs might play in human feeding. Stepping and crawling, as well as tongue movements, hand-to-mouth, and hand massage have only been identified in breastfeeding studies carried out in skin-to-skin contact.

In those existing studies, most of the researchers focused on neonatal, but not maternal, competence. Building upon Gunther's (1955) suggestions that mammalian mothers lie inert, the mothers studied were specifically directed not to touch their babies as part of the protocol. This design allowed researchers to demonstrate neonatal competence, suggesting that babies have an innate capacity to breastfeed, even without the mothers' assistance.

However, this design had some serious limitations in that it completely disregarded mothers and neglected to examine reciprocity or the critical interaction between the mother's and baby's innate abilities. Furthermore, the behaviours that were observed were attributed to the effects of skin-to-skin contact, not the mothers' and babies' positions or the impact of neonatal behavioural states. Paediatricians identified positions and behavioural states as the key variables releasing PNR activity (Amiel-Tison & Grenier, 1984; André-Thomas, Chesni, & Saint-Anne Dargassies, 1960; Brazelton & Nugent, 1995; Dubowitz, Dubowitz, & Mercuri, 1999; Prechtl, 1977). My prior study results concurred, identifying those two variables–positions and states–as related to the presence or absence and strength of response of PNRs.

Another reason to carry out descriptive, rather than experimental research concerns a more thorny issue. The English Medical Research Council (2000) highlights that descriptive studies supporting theoretical clarity are often omitted during the development of health interventions due to time and financial constraints. Many of the current protocols for assisting mothers to breastfeed were developed without proper evaluation and gold-standard evidence to support their effectiveness. We now know, and our low rates of breastfeeding continuance support this, that many of these techniques and procedures do not always work.

In the development of biological nurturing, it made scientific sense to try to avoid the same pitfalls. That is why I went back to the drawing board, selecting a descriptive-comparative design and a mixed-methods approach, enabling the systematic and objective identification of the different components of BN and how they interrelate. Nevertheless, it was also important to measure breastfeeding rates at both two and six weeks: not to find out cause-and-effect determinants, but to inform decisions about the feasibility of developing BN further as an intervention to support breastfeeding initiation. If the results showed that an equal number or fewer mothers were breastfeeding at these times than the UK national averages, then regardless of the findings for the mechanisms, the development of BN would be abandoned.

The immediate purpose of the PhD investigation, therefore, was not to test the effects of the BN intervention. Rather, it was to uncover the mechanisms of biological nurturing, establishing whether BN releases primitive neonatal reflexes as breastfeeding stimulants, as it appeared to do in my previous research. In addition, it was important to explore the overall contribution PNRs might make to infant feeding and to compare descriptions of any PNRs observed that appeared to stimulate feeding in both the bottle- and breastfeeding contexts.

When people undertake PhD research, there is a supervisory panel, and sometimes expert advisors, helping to maintain a high academic standard. For my study, both academic and clinical experts supported the work. The supervisory panel comprised a chairperson, two academic supervisors, and a clinical supervisor. A sub-group of breastfeeding experts was comprised of a lactation consultant/National Childbirth Trust breastfeeding counsellor, a La Leche League peer supporter, a cranial osteopath, and a consultant neonatologist.

A descriptive-comparative study design was selected, using a mixed-methods approach, with videotaped observations as the primary method of data collection. One session was filmed either in hospital or at home for both breast- and bottle-feeding mothers. In this book, we concentrate primarily on the findings for the breastfeeding group. A full description of the research design can be found in the thesis[3] and in a subsequent research article (Colson et al., 2008). However, the specific research questions and outcome measures are displayed in Table 1. This brief description of the objectives can help you understand the results.

---

3 The PhD thesis won the inaugural Royal College of Nursing Akinsanya award in 2006 and a bound copy is available for consultation in the Royal College of Nursing Library Steinberg Collection.

Research Questions and Outcome Measures

Table 1. Research Questions and Outcome Measures

Research Question	Outcome Measure
Can the components of BN be described? How do they interrelate and interact?	The description of the BN components and explanations for how they interact.
Does BN release PNRs? If so, how is BN influenced by the two key neurological variables: positions and states?	The identification and description of a number of PNRs as feeding stimulants across breastfeeding positions and neonatal behavioural states.
Can any PNRs be observed systematically to play a role in the feeding context?	Description of role, type, and potential function of PNRs
Should BN be developed further as an intervention to support breastfeeding?	Breastfeeding duration at two and six postnatal weeks

What About Skin-To-Skin Contact?

On the surface, mothers participating in BN show behaviours that are similar to those found in studies of Kangaroo Mother Care (KMC) (Anderson, 1989; Anderson et al., 2003; Ludington-Hoe & Galant, 1993). KMC is a method originally designed for pre-term infants where mothers incubate their nappy-clad babies in skin-to-skin contact. The baby lies prone on mother's chest, and this offers unrestricted access to the breast. At the time of my study, I was a fervent proponent of skin-to-skin contact. However, during the study, mothers on the postnatal ward often emphatically said that they did not want to undress. They also felt uncomfortable and worried about undressing their babies.

Although well-designed randomised controlled trials demonstrate a striking thermoregulatory benefit associated with skin-to skin contact, none of the babies under my charge was hypothermic, so I did not insist. Little by little, I paid increasing attention to mothers' comments. Research observations (Colson, 2000; Colson, 2002; Colson et al., 2003) suggested that, for any healthy baby, whether in skin-to-skin contact or lightly dressed, close juxtaposition with maternal-body contours, in full-frontal body contact was important for breastfeeding.

Interactions between the mother's and baby's bodies—whether or not there was skin-to-skin contact—appeared to stimulate a range of what appeared to be innate involuntary reflexes. Mouthing, licking, smelling, nuzzling, and nesting at the breast, crawling and rooting movements, searching and latching onto the breast, sucking and swallowing were commonly followed by sleeping, and then re-latching behaviours. In close body contact during episodes of biological nurturing, with or without skin-to-skin contact, mothers seemed to elicit these behaviours spontaneously. Maternal cues appeared to trigger babies' reflexes or baby cues released maternal responses. Together, these reciprocal behaviours appeared to aid breastfeeding initiation (Colson, 2000). I have included more details about these differences in Chapter 11.

Conclusion

Biological nurturing research did not end with the doctoral work exploring the mechanisms. Rather, the endpoint of research projects investigating biological nurturing is a reliable and valid intervention that supports breastfeeding initiation—and ultimately, this is my aim. In the case of BN, reliability means that two or more practitioners using BN would support the same mother in a similar way, making the same assessment of milk transfer. Validity means that the intervention enables mothers to breastfeed as they intend, taking into account that mothers' plans often change. For example, during pregnancy a mother may plan to mix feed. At birth, she may feel differently.

It is this incredible variety in perspective that makes it difficult to develop and assess an effective breastfeeding intervention. In fact, the development of any health intervention is complex, which is why the Medical Research Council (2000) provides specific guidance in this area. The Council defines a complex intervention as one where there are various inter-connecting parts or components that interrelate and interact to produce the desired effect. The challenge is to identify the active ingredients, or those components, that are essential to attain the expected outcome. The PhD study made an important contribution towards the achievement of that aim.

Chapter 5

The Components of
Biological Nurturing

Biological nurturing is a multifaceted, holistic intervention. We can talk about individual components, but to truly understand biological nurturing, you must recognise the synergistic relation between the components, and this relationship keeps changing. For in BN, as in other complex systems, the sum of the components is truly greater than the sum of the parts. This is because in BN, the sum of the components varies from mother to mother, so that all mothers and babies do not exhibit all of the innate behaviours, nor do these behaviours present in the same sequence. Rather, the mother's sequence of behaviours appears to be triggered by, and tailored to, the baby's needs.

The Components of Biological Nurturing Summarised

There were some real advantages to using a descriptive comparative design within a mixed-methods approach. BN could now be defined and the principal components summarised. The components are listed below and can be grouped and used to define BN as a collective term for positions, behaviours, and states that enhance breastfeeding initiation (Figure 4).

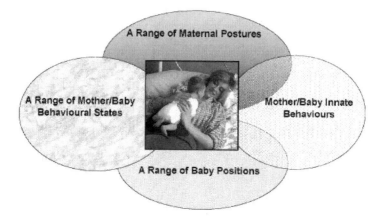

Figure 4. The Components of Biological Nurturing
Photo © Suzanne Colson.

In summary, the components comprise:

1. A range of maternal laid-back sitting postures or sacral sitting where the support from the bony pelvis is predominantly sacral rather than ischial.

2. A range of baby positions, including the direction of the baby's position or the neonatal lie (lying up and down, across, or obliquely on top of the mother's body).

3. Inborn neonatal reflexes and spontaneous maternal behaviours released by mother/baby positional interactions.

4. A range of neonatal and maternal behavioural states.

Figure 5 displays pictures of mothers illustrating the range of positions. Notice the body to body proximity: the babies' body curves are in close juxtaposition with the mothers' or with the environment.

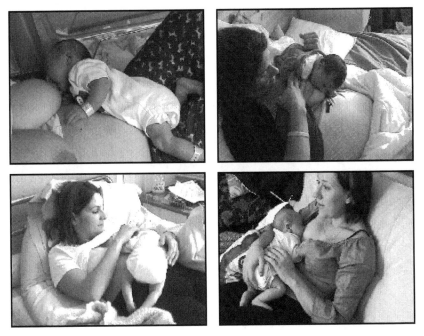

Figure 5. Biological Nurturing Positions

In the pictures, the maternal body takes the full weight of the baby, but in the picture in the upper right, the baby's feet, calves, and thighs are in close apposition with the bed. Photos © Suzanne Colson.

As Many Variables as There are Mothers

One aspect of BN that distinguishes it from previous approaches is the variability of each of its parts. The principle components–maternal postures and neonatal positions and the positional sub-components (neonatal lie within the positions and sacral sitting within the postures), together with the mother-baby behavioural states–are always present, but not held constant. Mothers' and babies' bodies are biologically designed to work together to ensure the survival of the species.

The Oxford dictionary defines a "mechanism" as *"a system of mutually adapted parts working together … a means by which a particular effect is produced"* (Thompson, 1995, p. 1728). Analysis revealed that laid-back sitting postures and neonatal frontal positions were the primary components of the *BN system*. Those two components were *"mutually adapted and working together"* to release innate behaviours. Friction, resulting from bodies brushing together, with gravity maintaining the baby in close frontal contact, were *the means* by which the *particular effect* or successful breastfeeding was *produced*. This is not really surprising as the laid-back maternal sitting posture used gravity positively, making it possible for every part of the baby's front to brush up against a maternal body contour or against part of the environment.

There will always be a range of baby positions and mother postures whose interactions release the reflexes as stimulants. This positional individuality promotes maternal comfort and releases pain-free effective latching and innate feeding behaviours. The range and variety in positions depend upon many factors, including the degree of privacy and anthropometric characteristics, such as the height of the mother and the weight and maturity of the baby.

When mothers are not taught a specific position, they often spontaneously use a degree of body slope that meets their needs at the time. This spontaneous degree of body slope appears to enhance eye-to-eye contact with the baby, without placing strain on the mother's neck. Biological nurturing appears to change breastfeeding into a two-way relationship characterised by reciprocity. The mechanisms are summarised in Table 2. Of all the mechanisms, the positive use of gravity is the most important. Note what this breastfeeding counsellor from Birmingham describes.

> *I notice that in BN the baby is most definitely "tummy to mummy" in all positions, as this is a fundamental part of releasing the reflexes to propel the baby toward the breast. I have seen this many times. In BN, the baby may be diagonal to the mother's body with bottom held by mother's hand, which falls naturally also in a diagonal position resting in her lap. A horizontal hold often seems rather uncomfortable. There appears to be a lot of research to support this BN view. I appreciate the mother's feeding position is different—being more laid-back.*

The next five chapters describe the individual components of BN along with the important role of gravity in greater detail. However, as described earlier, the real magic of BN occurs when the components work together.

Table 2. The Mechanisms of Biological Nurturing at a Glance

Biological Nurturing Laid-Back Maternal Sitting Postures:
Open the mother's body, increasing the dimensions of her torso.
Make the mother's frontal body region (part between the sternum and the pubis) available to the baby.
Encourage full frontal baby positions which release motor and other PNRs through body brushing.
Accommodate the baby's need to move towards a longitudinal or oblique lie.
Increase the number of approaches to the breast or the lie of the baby's position.
Work with (not against) gravitational forces.
Are fully supported, aiding relaxation and promoting freedom of movement.
Free mother's hands to groom and stroke.
Facilitate mother-baby gazing.
Promote maternal behaviours, protecting baby's breathing, thermoregulation and sleep.
Biological Nurturing Full-Frontal Baby Positions:
Require no back, head or neck pressure to keep the baby in place at the breast.
Facilitate self-attachment, although mothers guide, help, and assess baby's well-being.

Chapter 6

Primitive Neonatal Reflexes (PNRs)

People from many disciplines have shown a certain fascination with PNRs, from the early baby biographers, such as Darwin (1872) and Preyer (1893), to physicians, such as Peiper (1963), who catalogued more than 50 PNRs, making phylogenetic comparisons. Developmental psychologists, such as Piaget (1955), who was also a baby biographer, Illingworth (1963), and Gesell, Ilg, and Ames (1974) also introduced PNR assessments, using the work of well-known paediatricians. Indeed, in-depth understanding about PNRs comes from five landmark medical assessment instruments that were developed in the 1960s and 1970s (Amiel-Tison & Grenier, 1984; André-Thomas et al.,1960; Brazelton & Nugent, 1995; Dubowitz et al., 1999; Prechtl, 1977). These medical assessments integrated many PNRs as components of the neurological evaluation of the newborn baby. For example, the Brazelton and Nugent Neonatal Behavioral Assessment Scale (1995) evaluates 18 PNRs and is used by clinicians and researchers the world over.

Primitive neonatal reflexes are sometimes called archaic reflexes. Both expressions are collective terminology representing three kinds of innate movement: unconditioned reflexes, spontaneous reactions, and innate responses to environmental or endogenous stimuli. Together with infant state and tone, PNRs are used to map gestational age and to assess neurological function. For example, the Moro reflex, one of the first PNRs researchers documented, is probably the best known among health professionals. Parents may be more familiar with the stepping reflex, where the examiner, holding the baby around the chest, brushes the soles of the baby's feet against a hard surface. This releases automatic walking movements.

PNRs are simple reflexes supported by an intact nervous system. The medical evaluation also serves as a screening test. The strength and the absence of an expected PNR or the presence of one for longer than expected are considered predictors of concurrent neuropathology.

Successful feeding also depends upon an intact nervous system and three PNRs—rooting, sucking, and swallowing—are described formally as infant-feeding stimulants in the neonatal assessment instruments. More recently, several researchers, examining the effects of skin-to-skin contact, have introduced a potential feeding role for other PNRs. For example, Righard and

Frantz (1992) added hand-to-mouth and stepping and walking interpretations in the *Delivery Self-Attachment* video. Widstrom and colleagues (1987) named hand-to-mouth, stepping, and crawling reflexes, describing what they termed predictable behavioural patterns of how the baby held in skin-to-skin contact finds the breast during the first hour following birth. These patterns were then illustrated in a video called *Breastfeeding: The Baby's Choice* (Widstrom, 1996).

In the preterm context, brushing techniques are central to the release of rooting in the Newborn Individualized Developmental Care and Assessment Program (NIDCAP) developed by Als (1995) in the U.S. Nyqvist (2005) in Sweden lists "licking" as a developmental observation in the Preterm Infant Breastfeeding Behavior Scale (PIBBS). Results from the background studies articulating biological nurturing suggested that there were many more PNRs that might play a role in breastfeeding initiation and that skin-to-skin contact was not the independent variable.

Schools of Thought on Neurological Assessment

Different schools of thought inform the neurological assessment of the term and preterm infant. Each school draws upon Prechtl's (1977) extraordinary work giving detailed description of the PNRs and their releasers. However, there are four dominant and differing perspectives or neurological "world views" that underpin a philosophy of neonatal evaluation: *Le tonus*, or muscle-tone, paradigm developed by the French school (Amiel-Tison & Grenier, 1984) and the Dubowitz (1999) model in England; the reflexological approach developed by the Dutch school (Prechtl,1977); the behavioural-driven assessment developed by the American school (Brazelton & Nugent, 1995); and Prechtl's (2001) relatively new ontogenetic-adaptation paradigm, where general neonatal movements (GMs) are observed and interpreted as predictors of long-term neurological outcomes.

PNRs are weakly present by 28 completed weeks of gestation, and the strength of PNR response is a major predictor of maturation (Dubowitz et al., 1999). The Dubowitz (1999) model focuses, for the most part, upon prematurity, and the stick figures of babies in flexion and extension are recognised the world over.

Gestational age, neonatal positions, and neonatal behavioural states are the variables that have been shown to influence the qualitative expression, defined as the simple presence or absence of PNRs, and their strength of reaction or response. Equipped with this knowledge, Prechtl (1977), in landmark work studying over 1,500 babies, standardised the evaluation techniques and scoring procedures used during the neonatal evaluation. Each reflex was described and the procedures and techniques for its release minutely detailed, and these were understandably inflexible. Two examiners assessing the same baby would need to attain the same result, as the examination was designed to detect pathology versus well being. The assessment literally said, "yeah or nay" to nervous-system function. Therefore, to achieve high inter-assessor reliability, Prechtl standardised everything, including the height of the examination table and the lighting and heating in the room. He defined neonatal behavioural states and those examination positions that would release optimal PNR responses. That is why most of the PNRs are released and assessed when the baby is in a quiet alert behavioural state, even though PNRs can often be observed in sleep states.

The Impact of Neonatal Position

Three neonatal positions are used by pediatricians to release the reflexes: supine, prone, and a position called ventral suspension, where the examiner holds the baby around the thorax with feet dangling. Finger and plantar grasping, sucking, rooting, and the Babinski reflex, a kind of a toe fanning response, are among those examined when babies are supine. When babies lie prone, such responses as spontaneous head righting, head lifting, and crawling are released. In ventral suspension, automatic stepping and placing are triggered. Placing is described as a lifting and placing movement in response to brushing the top of the baby's foot against a hard surface, usually the examination table.

What Do PNRs Have to Do with Breastfeeding?

People are often puzzled, wondering what such movements as placing, finger or plantar grasping, or a Babinski toe fan could possibly have to do with infant feeding. For the answers to these questions, we need to look more closely at biological nurturing.

The overall purpose of my PhD study was to investigate primitive neonatal reflexes as the primary mechanisms of biological nurturing. Having observed PNR-like movements appearing to stimulate feeding during episodes of BN and because all healthy normal babies have these reflexes at birth, I thought that increased understanding of these inborn movements might yield further knowledge about how best to support breastfeeding initiation for healthy term babies.

Primitive Neonatal Reflexes: Number and Classification

In my study, 54 mother-baby pairs were videotaped and studied, 40 in the breastfeeding group and 14 in the bottle-feeding group. Twenty PNRs were identified, described, compared, and validated in the feeding context with high (0.8) inter-rater agreement. PNRs were categorised into four types: endogenous, rhythmic, motor, and anti-gravity. Three feeding functions were suggested: cueing, searching or finding PNRs, and those which appeared to help sustain milk transfer. The PNRs together with the type and function are displayed in Figure 6.

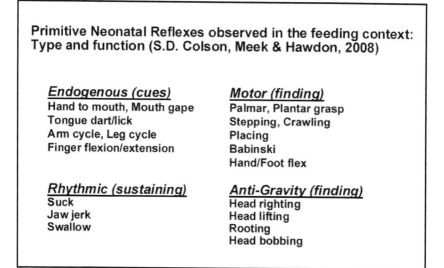

Figure 6.

The Role Played By PNRs: Unexpected Findings

We never imagined that PNRs could have a negative role in the feeding context. Yet time and again, we saw reflexes pushing the baby away from the breast. Jerky movements, head shaking, leg scrambling, body flinging, arm thrashing, fighting, scratching, leg cycling movements that looked like kicking … we never anticipated such description. On the other hand, we sometimes observed the same movements as smooth and coordinated. In other words, the same reflexes looked like they could either help the baby find the breast, latch on, and sustain milk transfer–or they appeared to thwart latching and successful breastfeeding.

Researchers have always described the rooting and sucking reflexes as feeding stimulants. Therefore, this dual role that the PNRs appeared to play caught us by surprise. At the same time, during data analysis, the mother's breastfeeding position emerged as unquestionably the single most important variable, either releasing the reflexes as stimulants or as breastfeeding barriers. As a result, we needed to formulate research definitions to describe a range of maternal breastfeeding postures in a systematic and objective fashion. These definitions will be illustrated and discussed in chapter 7. In that chapter, we also explore the postural causes of this dual role explaining how an inborn reflex response like rooting, which is "normally" supposed to stimulate latch, could be transformed into a negative influence resulting in latch failure.

Latch Failure

Consecutive UK feeding surveys characterise latch failure either as "fighting the breast" or as "breast refusal", where a baby who should be hungry is too sleepy to latch or fails to suck (Bolling, Grant, Hamlyn & Thornton, 2007; Foster, Lader, & Cheesbrough, 1997; Hamlyn, Brooker, Oleinikova, & Wands, 2002; Martin & Monk, 1982; Martin & White, 1987; White, Freeth & O'Brien, 1992). Objective descriptions of what is visible or audible, however, are sparse. Gohil (2006), an Indian paediatrician, offers a vivid description of what he calls a new breastfeeding behaviour observed during engorgement. Termed "breast boxing", he describes some PNR-like movements associated with latch failure that we often observed in my study.

> *It was observed that the infant does not suckle and pushes himself away with his fisted hands at the breasts or abdomen of the mother, and kicks away at the mother's abdomen and avoids feeding* (Gohil, 2006, p. 268).

Our data suggested that these kicking and pushing away behaviours were often combined with increasingly frenetic activity and to-and-fro horizontal head shaking, thwarting latch. Typically, the baby was in a quiet alert state at the start of the feed and after about a minute, when latch was not successful, side-to-side head rooting movements increased in frequency and intensity. These were often accompanied by the hand-to-mouth reflex, where the hungry baby appeared to prefer sucking on his fist instead of the breast.

The Baby Friendly Initiative (BFI) (UNICEF, 2010; WHO, 1997 p. 94) discusses latch refusal, suggesting that mothers often interpret these head shaking movements as the baby "saying no" to breastfeeding. At the first videotaped episode in my study, over half the breastfed babies displayed these negative behaviours, preventing them from latching. The BFI is quick to reassure that, contrary to maternal interpretation, this is "normal behaviour"—and I agree with this point. Rooting is often characterised by a range of movement (lip twitches to exaggerated side-to-side head shaking); the hand-to-mouth reflex and arm and leg cycling are an integral part of the "normal" behavioural repertoire of the neonate. However, we observed systematically that, in certain positional situations, these inborn movements appear to be obstructive due to gravity. In certain positions, the force of gravity appeared to pull the mothers and babies apart and override what might be considered the normal nature of the reflex response in the feeding context.

How Does Position Affect the Role of the Reflexes

Those mothers experiencing the negative PNR effects were either lying on their sides or sitting upright, bolt upright, or leaning slightly forward, as they had been taught. Upright mothers often placed the baby on a pillow in front of and at right angles to their bodies, and although the baby was often "tummy to mummy", there was usually a gap or angle between the mother's and baby's bodies. The baby's thighs, calves, and feet were often in contact with thin air. Importantly, mothers *had to hold* their babies in positions where they applied pressure along the baby's back to keep him on the pillow and/or at breast level. I have termed this *dorsal feeding*. The more the mother struggled to elicit mouth gape, leading in with the chin, the tighter she gripped the baby's back. This firm grip often extended to the baby's neck or head. The firmer the grip, the more the baby struggled with frantic arm and/or leg cycles, increasing in strength and amplitude as the baby worked himself up to a crying state.

Dorsal Feeding

Peiper (1963) compares and contrasts positional phenomenon across species, assuming that dorsal feeding (where mothers must physically hold their babies' back) is uniquely human. In fact, we have always believed that our babies, unlike some of our mammalian cousins, are obligate dorsal feeders (i.e., need to feed with pressure on their backs). Whether breast- or bottle-feeding, a baby who is an obligate dorsal feeder always needs back pressure to maintain positional stability and to keep the baby at breast level, no matter if the mother is sitting upright or lying on her side. You can see how human mothers need to hold their babies, applying this pressure down the baby's back, in Figure 7.

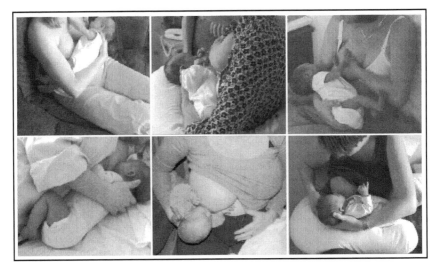

Figure 7. Dorsal Breastfeeding Positions

This figure illustrates dorsal feeding across the range of well-known baby holding techniques: clutch or rugby/football hold, cradle and cross cradle hold, and side-lying. Middle photo lower row © Trix Simmons; other photos © Suzanne Colson.

Frontal Feeding

In contrast, my research on biological nurturing positions found that human babies may breastfeed best when they are not in the traditional holds where mothers must apply back and/or neck pressure. As soon as mothers laid back, and only three mothers did this spontaneously in the first videotaped episode, their babies were immediately in what Peiper (1963) termed a full abdominal position. I refer to this as a frontal-feeding position. In these full chest and tummy positions, another baby reflex was observed, a pendular or head bobbing movement, which appeared to be released from a fixed point in the baby's spine. This movement was also documented previously by Scheildt and Prechtl (1951) (in Peiper, 1963), who suggested that vertical pendular movements stimulate latching in non-human, abdominal-feeding mammals. This includes animals, such as puppies and hamsters, where the baby's tummy hugs the ground when they feed.

I termed this position "frontal feeding" because observations suggested that it was not just the abdomen that was involved. The entire frontal region of the body, comprising the chest area, as well as the abdomen was implicated. For our purposes, this region extends from the sternum to the pubic bone. In full frontal positions, the baby's thighs, calves, and feet tops were spontaneously applied either to the mother's body or to a part of the environment (the bed, sofa, chair, bed clothes, etc.).

Babies in frontal feeding positions latched on quicker and easier, and they also had some common points. First, their mothers were laid back, but not all to the same degree of body slope. Second, the baby was neither held vertically nor parallel to the mother's body. Rather he positioned himself lying longitudinally (up and down) or obliquely, on top of the mother. In other words, the baby always lay prone, but importantly slanted upward, with a natural physiological body tilt. This upward tilt was due to the gradient provided by the gentle maternal body slope.

The frontal feeding baby often approached the breast using the pendular head-bobbing reflex, which involved the entire trigeminal area. Importantly, mothers did not have to hold the baby: no back, neck, or head pressure was required or necessary to achieve positional stability or to maintain the baby at breast level. Instead, gravitational forces helped to keep the baby on the mother's body. Gravity also appeared to make the reflexes smoother and more coordinated, aiding latch and sustaining milk transfer, as Nikki Lee, an American lactation consultant, describes below.

> *Dear Suzanne:*
>
> *I have integrated [biological nurturing] into my 18-Hour Interdisciplinary Breastfeeding Management Course for the US. I show pictures from your article and discuss laid-back breastfeeding. I show the video clip about infant reflexes that can either help or hinder breastfeeding. Almost everyone can recognize the baby with the frantic arm and leg cycling and is very impressed with the change once the mother lays-back. I shudder to remember how many babies whose legs and arms I held tightly so a mother could breastfeed....we learn and grow, thank goodness!!*
>
> *Another thing; when I worked in labor and delivery and postpartum, I would see babies doing that "playing" at the breast. They would root and root and root and not latch on. I thought it was an impact of the epidural!! Thank you for your wonderful work.*

Andrea, a breastfeeding counsellor from the UK, described her personal experiences with her first baby, and how health professionals misunderstood the PNRs her baby was exhibiting.

> *Dear Suzanne,*
>
> *It was so lovely meeting you at the weekend......I just wanted to share my own experience with you. When my first daughter was born (nearly 8 years ago), I breastfed her in a sitting position (as been told and taught) but was never able to put her down afterwards without her waking and screaming. So we came to the agreement (me and her) that I would start feeding her in a nearly sitting up position and then gradually slouch back (till reaching BN position), which would leave us*

both happy. After a feed she would wiggle herself into a nice position and would sleep or just watch the world go by.

One day, just after such a feed the midwife came to see me. Jana (my daughter) lifted her head to see what was happening and the midwife said straight away "Don't let her do that, she will damage her neck."

A few weeks later I had my check up at the GP and Jana was screaming her head off when I laid down on the examination bench. So I said to the GP, I will just hold her will you get on with the examination (to the GP's dismay). I put Jana on my tummy (having propped myself up as much as I could) and she was lifting her head to see where she was. Again the GP said "She will damage her neck if she lifts her head so high. Don't encourage it. You are spoiling her if you always hold her." I was in tears afterwards till I spoke to my own mother who simply smiled and said "that's what they told me as well. Just ignore it, go with your instincts and if any professional challenges you, well, tell them what they want to hear. It makes your life easier, but in our family no one has let their babies cry and they all turned out well."

I can't believe, that just 8 years ago they actively discouraged headbobbing, etc.

The common components of each approach are compared and contrasted in Table 3.

Table 3. Primitive Neonatal Reflexes Released in Upright vs. Laid-back Mother Postures

Latch Refusal or Breast Fighting	Easy and Effective Latch
Mother sits bolt upright with lap at right angles to back or leans slightly forward.	Mother leans back at different degrees of body slope; not lying flat on her back or on her side.
Mother's head, neck, and shoulders are not supported and her shoulders are often unbalanced and/or hunched.	Maternal body has the potential for complete support including head, neck, shoulders, upper back, lower back, and legs.
One maternal forearm and hand must hold the baby; the other hand often holds the breast.	Mother has at least one hand free; often both hands are free. Maternal arms often lie lightly on or loosely encircling the baby.
Mother must hold her baby applying back pressure; this pressure often extends to the baby's neck or head.	There is no need to hold the baby, but sometimes the baby's head rests on mother's arms or in her hands.
Baby is held in one of three ways: cradle, cross cradle, or rugby/football hold.	There are potentially 360 baby positions and no standard holds.
There is a pre-determined way to approach the breast; baby held at breast level must approach the breast from below.	Like the hands of a clock, the baby can approach the breast from any angle, i.e., from above or below the breast.
Baby lies "tummy to/facing mummy", but there is often a gap or angle formed between the mother's and baby's bodies.	Baby lies tummy on mummy with no gap or angle between baby's and mother's bodies.
Baby lies vertically parallel or at right angles to the mother's body transversely across her midriff.	Baby sometimes lies on top and across the mother's body, but usually lies on top longitudinally or obliquely.
Baby's legs and feet are either loosely or poorly applied to mother's body; often only in contact with thin air.	Baby's thighs, calves, feet tops, and soles are touching & closely applied to the maternal body, the furniture, or bed clothes, etc.
The first point of breast contact is the chin; baby's mouth gapes wide and lower lip is below lower half of the areola.	The first point of breast contact often involves the entire Trigeminal area, with symmetrical mouth gape and attachment.
Mothers often latch or attach the baby onto the breast.	Babies often self attach.

Reflex Activity or Hunger and Interest?

Hunger and interest are common watchwords characterising breastfeeding initiation. Faced with latch failure, health professionals and mothers alike often say that the baby is either not hungry or not interested in breastfeeding. In view of the strong reflex component stimulating breastfeeding observed during episodes of biological nurturing, we must address these interpretations.

The Role of Hunger in Frontal Feeding

First, hunger is not the only neonatal drive to breastfeed. Let us recall that healthy term infants are born well-fed, and during the first 24 hours, they only ingest small amounts of milk (Hartmann, 1987). This is not to suggest that hunger does not regulate feeding behaviours, rather I suggest that babies latch on and breastfeed for a variety of reasons in different situations.

Babies who remain lying prone, but at a physiological body tilt upwards on top of their mother's body, go in and out of drowsy and sleep states. In my study, compelling video data show how they often latch on or re-latch whilst asleep, even after 30 or 45 minutes of good milk transfer characterised by sucking bursts and audible swallowing. Independent of hunger, babies will often latch again and again in response to positional stimuli releasing feeding reflexes.

The BN approach helps to condition the reflexes earlier. During the first days, the baby is learning how to coordinate suck and swallow with breathing for the first time. When the healthy term baby is in the right habitat, it usually does not take long to achieve reflex conditioning and physiological coordination, suggesting that this is best done before maternal milk volume increases (approximately the third postnatal day) and hunger increasingly becomes a factor.

Likewise, biological nurturing research rejects the common notion that the baby is not interested in breastfeeding to explain latch reluctance or failure. One way to trigger a latch is by releasing the foot reflexes, such as the Babinski and plantar grasp. This strong foot-to-mouth association was fascinating to observe. For example, when mothers wanted to put their sleeping babies down, they often checked to see if the baby was finished by spontaneously stroking the baby's feet. Of course, this was easy to do; they usually had both hands free because they did not need to hold the baby.

Neonatal interest can be defined as the amount of time during which the baby has focused attention on a stimulus (Brazelton & Nugent, 1995). "Interest", therefore, can only occur during a quiet alert behavioural state, for example, when the baby looks at bright lights or tracks bright objects, like a red ball, with his eyes, or gazes intently upon his mother's face. During the first three postnatal days, these times of focused attention are precious, promoting reciprocal behaviours, like mimicry and mutual sensorial discovery and communication. Babies are known to spend 75% to 80% of their time sleeping, moving rapidly from one state to the next, so that comparatively these quiet alert times do not last very long during the first three postnatal days.

These facts suggest that "interest in breastfeeding" is probably not the right turn of phrase. Furthermore, when health professionals suggest that the baby is "not interested" in breastfeeding, it can undermine a mother's confidence, making her think that the baby does not like her milk or that she does not have enough. This can lead to feelings of guilt and inadequacy, which are heightened when the baby rapidly glugs the artificial milk drink in the bottle that is often given to the baby who is "disinterested" in breastfeeding. This rapid deglutition usually has nothing to do with interest or hunger, but rather occurs because the length of the bottle teat is specifically designed to release the suck reflex. A suck then releases a swallow. The baby held in a dorsal feeding position is boxed in by maternal body, arms, and bottle; he usually has no choice but to suck. He ingests the milk rapidly because the reflexes have been released, not necessarily because he is hungry or interested. We know that the newborn's stomach capacity is small, holding about 30 mls, or less than an ounce. Yet fifteen minutes later, when the baby brings up a large quantity of milk, no one associates this output with the "forced" bottle-feeding. Instead, the 60 mls ingested is the index used to measure feeding success, even though this amount compared to neonatal stomach capacity indicates that the baby has been overfed. Taken together, these facts and observations lead us to suggest that the mechanisms underpinning breastfeeding initiation during the first days are simple reflex activity, not always triggered or associated with hunger and interest.

An example can help to clarify the misunderstanding about eliciting a reflex versus interest. The knee-jerk reflex is a simple response mediated in the spinal cord and similar to many PNRs. The knee jerk is also used as a screening test to assess neurological function across the life span. When a doctor, using a patella hammer, attempts to elicit the knee-jerk reflex and the knee does not respond, he does not suggest that it is because the knee is "not interested" in jerking. The doctor also does not suggest waiting three hours to try again!

All nurses know that simple reflexes are assessed across behavioural states. For example, nurses are taught how to assess reflex activity in the unconscious patient. In the same way, when babies are in light sleep and drowsy states, the inevitable body brushing releases the motor and searching PNRs. When the baby is sleeping, the reflex actions releasing self-attachment are somewhat blunted, reducing the strength of the response. Nevertheless, these mechanisms produce latch, just as the doctor using the patellar hammer produces the knee jerk.

In addition, we can certainly state that "interest" is not central to a successful transition from foetus to neonate. However, what is absolutely fundamental is early and frequent suckling during the first three days. Early and frequent suckling ensures a successful postnatal adaptation for healthy term babies. Early and frequent suckling keeps the baby in the normal habitat, protects the baby against infection, keeps him warm, and ensures the tactile, olfactory, and eye-to-eye contact crucial to brain development (Bergman, 2010;

Odent, 2002). Early and frequent suckling helps to maintain blood glucose concentrations at just the right levels. As described earlier, metabolically, when babies breastfeed frequently, they generate ketone bodies, an alternative source of fuel for the neonatal brain (Hawdon et al., 1992). Research clearly demonstrates that the earlier babies latch on and suckle, the easier it is to establish breastfeeding (Riordan & Hoover, 2010).

If early breastfeeding initiation has to do with releasing and conditioning reflexes—as the biological nurturing research data suggest—then we must consider eliminating the words "interest and hunger" from our vocabulary during the time of breastfeeding initiation.

Chapter 7

Mother's Breastfeeding Posture

Who would have ever imagined that the position the mother sits in–mother's breastfeeding posture–would be central to the release of the PNRs as stimulants? Yet, that is what our observations suggested. Once we realised this, we needed to come up with a whole new set of research definitions.

Operational definitions are those used during a research investigation. These definitions are usually predetermined, enhancing objectivity and reliability of description. In the PhD study, however, the flexibility inherent in the descriptive design made it possible to identify and operationalise other ingredients or components identified at any time during the investigation. This enabled us to describe and define an unanticipated versatility in maternal breastfeeding positions.

We, therefore, spent hours studying the video clips, using both slow/fast motion and pausing techniques to capture still pictures. Luckily, two members of the PhD expert group had specialised knowledge from other disciplines. The NCT lactation consultant was originally qualified as a structural engineer and the cranial osteopath was trained to make fine calculations comparing anatomical structures. In consultation with the supervisory panel, it was therefore possible to formulate, in retrospect, approximate but concrete and measurable angles of maternal body slope, quantifying a range of maternal postures.

New Angles on Breastfeeding

The baby's position at the breast is currently believed to be the single most important variable associated with the quest for "the correct latch", enabling pain-free, effective breastfeeding (Renfrew, Woolridge, & McGill, 2000; Renfrew et al., 2005). The difference between breast positioning and breast attachment has been clarified in the literature (Inch, 2003). Although it is clear that these terms refer to the neonate, confusion can result from using the word "position" for both mother and baby. Therefore, we used the word "posture" to refer to the mother's position, whereas the word "position" always referred to the baby.

For the breastfeeding mothers who experienced latch refusal, sore nipples, or any other problems during the videotaped session, baby positions and postural changes were suggested after about five minutes, and the videotape captured both before and after episodes. When we compared these episodes, we found striking differences in anatomical postural support. To clarify these differences, we need to look at the bony pelvis.

The Role of the Bony Pelvis

Kapandji (1974), a French orthopaedic surgeon, integrated and illustrated complex physiology and mechanical functioning of joints and muscles within the anatomical context. His explanations and illustrations, together with those from recent English midwifery textbooks, provide the basis for understanding the difference between upright and laid-back sitting postures (see textbox).

The Bony Pelvis

The bony pelvis is literally a pivotal system supporting the abdomen. It houses the reproductive organs and links the vertebral column to the legs (Kapandji, 1974). Transmitting gravitational forces from the vertebral column to the lower limbs, the pelvis comprises four bony parts and three joints: two sacro-iliac and the symphysis pubis joint (Kapandji, 1974). The coccyx, the lowest part of the spine, articulates with the sacrum, a triangular-shaped bone composed of five fused sacral vertebrae vertically wedged between two iliac bones, sometimes called innominate bones, which are paired and symmetrical (Kapandji, 1974).

The iliac bones comprise three parts: the ilia or wing-like upper crests, which extend to and fuse with the pubis, thus forming two-fifths of the upper border of the acetabulum, the point of femoral articulation. The ischia, each extending from the acetabulum above, form a downward projection or protuberance of rounded bony mass below, called ischial tuberosities. The pubis is a small bone linking the ilia, anteriorly, and forming one-fifth of the anterior acetabulum (Henderson & MacDonald, 2004; Kapandji, 1974).

The sacrum, suspended from the iliac bones by ligaments, forms "a self locking system", whereby the greater the weight, the more tightly it locks (Kapandji, 1974, p. 56). Figure 8 illustrates these parts of the bony pelvis. Sacral movement is achieved through the sacro-iliac joints with a relatively limited range. Sacral nutation, coming from the Latin nutare, meaning to nod, refers to a complex system of sacral forward and backward rotational movements (Kapandji, 1974). Figure 9 illustrates sacral rotation.

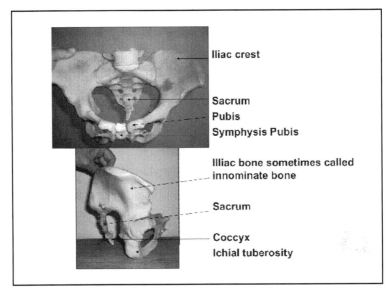

Iliac crest

Sacrum
Pubis
Symphysis Pubis

Illiac bone sometimes called
innominate bone

Sacrum

Coccyx
Ichial tuberosity

Figure 8. The Bony Pelvis
Photos © Suzanne Colson.

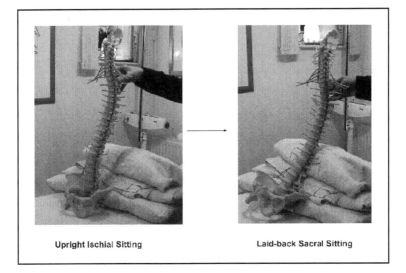

Upright Ischial Sitting   Laid-back Sacral Sitting

Figure 9. Sacral Nutation
Photos © Suzanne Colson.

Pelvic Sitting Support

When sitting upright or leaning slightly forward, the body mass is supported evenly by the two ischial tuberosities. In ischial sitting postures, for example, those used to drive a car, ride a bike, or work at the computer, the weight of the trunk sits firmly upon a solid base, either a chair or a seat (Kapandji, 1974). Strictly speaking, it is irrelevant if the base has a back since a chair back only limits the potential to recline. However, having a back support may add feelings of security (Kapandji, 1974). Body weight is placed equally on both ischial tuberosities if the seat is at a height that permits the thighs to be parallel to the floor and the feet to rest flat on the floor. The body leans forward from the hips when necessary, but does not curve at shoulders or neck (Kapandji, 1974).

This is the sitting posture that is normally termed "correct". The body is aligned from the hips up, just as when standing "correctly". Interestingly, Kapandji (1974, p. 112) calls this "correct" postural position, the "typist position", characterising it as fraught with potential for muscular fatigue and the most difficult body posture to sustain.

In contrast, when sitting laid back, for example, sprawled on a chair or sofa while watching television, the back of the chair or sofa always supports the body. Bony pelvic reliance comprises the posterior surface of the sacrum and the coccyx with limited ischial support (Kapandji, 1974). Kapandji (1974, p. 112) terms this posture the "position of relaxation". It is neither sitting nor lying, but is "achieved with the help of cushions or specially designed chairs". Figure 10 compares and contrasts bony pelvic reliance, picturing an adaptation of Kapandji's "typist's position" with his "position of relaxation".

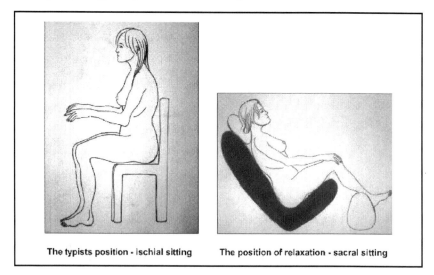

The typists position - ischial sitting   The position of relaxation - sacral sitting

Line drawings © Ken Tackett. Adapted from Kapandji, 1974.

Having understood these bony postural facts, and the small but important range of potential maternal pelvic movement, it became straightforward to define maternal posture using three parameters: degree of recline or body slope, bony pelvic reliance, and body support. Definitions determining the scientific angle of recline are summarised in Figure 11, and the operational definitions used during the PhD study are shown in Table 4.

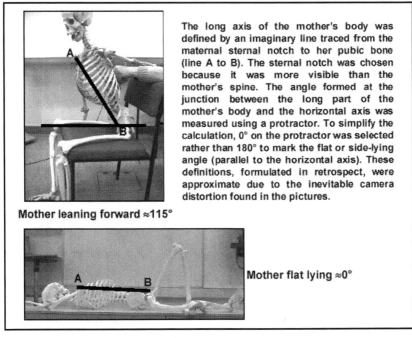

The long axis of the mother's body was defined by an imaginary line traced from the maternal sternal notch to her pubic bone (line A to B). The sternal notch was chosen because it was more visible than the mother's spine. The angle formed at the junction between the long part of the mother's body and the horizontal axis was measured using a protractor. To simplify the calculation, 0° on the protractor was selected rather than 180° to mark the flat or side-lying angle (parallel to the horizontal axis). These definitions, formulated in retrospect, were approximate due to the inevitable camera distortion found in the pictures.

Mother leaning forward ≈115°

Mother flat lying ≈0°

Figure 11. Calculating the angle of recline
Photos © Suzanne Colson.

Table 4. Operational Definition for Maternal Posture

	Degree of Recline	Bony Pelvic Reliance	Body Support
Upright Sitting	>74°	Ischial	Head, neck, shoulders, upper back lightly touching or not touching seat back
Laid-Back Sitting	15° to 74°	Sacral	Head, neck, upper back firmly against seat back
Flat/Side Lying	0° to 14°	None	Head, neck, torso against bed

Figure 12 illustrates these definitions in the flesh. Observe how the bottle-feeding mother on the left is ischial sitting, upright at 90°, as is the breastfeeding mother in the middle. On the right, the same breastfeeding mother has changed to sacral sitting and is semi-reclined at a 35° angle.

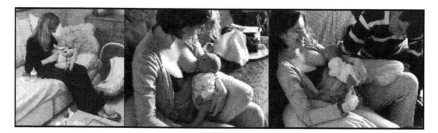

Figure 12.
Photos © Suzanne Colson.

Postures and Breastfeeding Duration: Results of Our Study

The 40 mothers in the breastfeeding group tried out biological nurturing in a variety of maternal body slope (at least on one occasion, at videotaping). At six postnatal weeks, all were breastfeeding–87.5% (n=35) exclusively. The 100% rate of breastfeeding duration occurred despite over a quarter of the mothers (n=11) having a caesarean birth. These results need to be interpreted with caution, as some would suggest that they imply cause and effect, whereas there is no such intent as discussed previously.

Other factors could also account for increased breastfeeding rates. First, a breastfeeding assessment was carried out by whoever was present. Mothers self reported, partners, and parents commented validating the experience.

I was only present as an observer and a research midwife; however, access to the various hospitals had been negotiated with the view that mothers and babies would remain safe under my care. I made professional evaluations of latch and milk transfer, although these were only shared verbally with the mother if and when needed. Nevertheless, I hold strong beliefs in every mother's capacity to breastfeed. Perhaps my convictions were transmitted in tacit ways, and we must ask the question: Can the beliefs and attitudes of the health professional affect breastfeeding outcomes? My personal convictions may have influenced the mothers. Some would suggest that this personal component is integral to breastfeeding support and is just as important as any other ingredient of an intervention.

A key finding was that more PNRs were observed as breastfeeding stimulants, aiding latch and sustaining milk transfer, when mothers sat laid-back than when they sat upright or lay on their sides, and this difference was statistically significant (Colson et al., 2008).

Mother Postures at the First Videotaped Episode

Three mothers spontaneously used laid-back sitting postures. A fourth mother wanted to be filmed trying out breastfeeding, like in the *Delivery, Self Attachment* video (Righard & Frantz, 1992), which meant that she was also laid-back during the first episode. Towards the end of the study, five mothers shared their problems with me before I filmed them and, having understood the central role played by maternal posture, I suggested that they might try laid-back postures during the filming. This meant that 9 of the 40 breastfeeding mothers were filmed laid-back right from the first episode. Those nine mothers experienced pain-free effective breastfeeding, five for the first time. Problems such as sore nipples (n=3), back ache (n=1), and latch refusal (n=1) were immediately improved.

Does This Mean That Mothers Should Never Initiate Breastfeeding in Upright Postures?

Human mothers and babies are extremely versatile, able to breastfeed in many different positions, and it would not be helpful to prescribe laid-back postures as the only way to initiate breastfeeding. Observations for the first episode demonstrated that 12 of the 27 breastfeeding mothers who sat upright latched their baby successfully onto the breast with good milk transfer. However, only a quarter of them (n=3) were pain-free; the other nine mothers modified their baby's positions, their own postures, or both in subsequent episodes to achieve an increase in comfort.

Likewise, three of the four mothers who started the feed lying on their sides latched the baby successfully with good milk transfer. However, side-lying was not sustainable for two of the four mothers who subsequently changed posture: one said she had sore nipples and another said she had back ache. That meant that 11 mothers (over 25% of the sample) breastfed through pain during the first episode. These findings replicate Sulcova's observations of postural discomfort.

The mother who wanted to try out breastfeeding in skin-to-skin contact and using the positions she saw in the *Delivery and Self Attachment* video was an experienced breastfeeding mother having her second baby. Following a home birth, she had no breastfeeding difficulties. Interestingly, she had seen the videotape (Righard & Frantz, 1992) some years prior to this pregnancy, but had never tried it out. She expressed a desire to try the flat-lying postures to see if the baby would self-attach (like the ones in the videotape). Her baby did, in fact, self-attach, but she is recorded on the research videotape saying that she prefers upright sitting. However, following completion of the postnatal questionnaire (at six weeks), she subsequently sent me a personal VHS videotape, recorded by her husband, demonstrating how her baby in full BN baby positions and flat-lying mother postures, self-attached, indicating that she had tried this again. I feel that her initial experience needs to be registered, as she was the only mother who, having tried more reclined postures, is recorded to prefer being upright.

Below are some questions I have received on the issue of traditional breastfeeding positions versus BN.

Hi Suzanne

I am a Student Breastfeeding Counsellor and have been following and researching your work on BN for a few months now….. I just wondered what you think BN means for more traditional positions, and is there a place for both or do you think BN is the ultimate way forward? As a student BFC who will be helping women in the future, I just want to figure out what BN means for me and the way I "teach" in the future.

Hi Claire,

I think that mothers and babies are extremely versatile, able to breastfeed in a variety of positions, and this is perhaps what makes us different from other mammals. Nevertheless, I wonder if BN maternal positions are more species specific, in that the amount of body space available to accommodate the movements of the neonate is increased when mother leans back. In traditional positions, the baby usually lies across the midriff because the body is closed, whereas in BN babies lie longitudinally or obliquely. We have a relatively small midriff compared to say a polar bear, whose babies often feed vertically, but polar bears also use a variety of positions.

❦

Dear Suzanne,

I am a student BFC with the NCT. A question that I didn't have the opportunity to ask after your presentation: do you find that babies who are started on breastfeeding along biological nurturing lines, go on to feed in more "conventional" positions, lying across the mother's lap, for example? I sort of presumed that once they'd been allowed to find the nipple and initiate breastfeeding on their own natural terms, they would later be more flexible about different positions, but I'd be really interested to know if this is so. I would love to teach couples about this approach to breastfeeding, but I can already hear women telling me that they want to be able to feed their babies while out and about, and it's very hard to recline comfortably on a park bench or cafe chair!

Dear Ellie,

Thank you for your kind words. I really enjoyed the conference and talking with all the NCT mothers. Itdoesnottakelongforthereflexestobecomeconditionedand thenmothersuseavarietyofpositions.Sometimestheylean backjustabitwhentheyareoutasmanyfindthiscomfortable. BN maternal postures can be more upright and still use gravity positively. It is just when mothers are bolt upright that gravity often works against latch. Nevertheless, once the reflexes are conditioned, it usually does not make any difference at all. When mothers are out and about, they can use any position that is comfortable. Sotheanswertoyourquestionisyes,mothersdonothaveto reclinewhentheyareout,andtheolderbabywilljustlatch, even if a mother is upright, when reflexes are conditioned.

Dear Suzanne,

Thank you so much for getting back to me so swiftly! I'm very encouraged by what you've said—it makes sense that babies adapt to different positions once they've established breastfeeding, I suppose. It doesn't make evolutional sense to be too inflexible, after all. I was really so struck by BN, and can't wait to try it out myself, but knew that mothers would want to know how it worked for them after the first early weeks. Thank you again,

Ellie

In summary, posture is a dynamic variable, changing often to enhance enjoyment and meet our needs no matter what we are doing. There is a strong argument suggesting that people will continue to do the things they enjoy, and this makes maternal comfort during breastfeeding a key issue in breastfeeding duration.

Maternal Comfort Mechanisms

All mothers experience a wide range of challenges to their personal comfort right after birth. The abrupt change in body shape can be a real shock, and sometimes body parts feel sensitive, ache, or are sore. This can be compounded by abdominal pain if the mother has had a caesarean birth, or perineal pain if she has had an episiotomy or an operative or assisted delivery. Breastfeeding often exacerbates discomfort as breasts and nipples can hurt, and many mothers complain of neck tension and shoulder pain, as it is difficult to maintain the "typist position" for long periods of time.

Laid-back breastfeeding, by definition, means that every part of the mother's body–importantly, her head, neck, shoulders, and upper and lower back are relaxed. Mothers often say that as soon as they sit back, the shoulder and neck tension melt away. Nipple pain is often alleviated immediately, and this may happen because gravity is not dragging the baby down the upright maternal midriff. Mothers also have increased freedom of movement, as one or both hands are free; their bodies hold the baby, not their arms. Figure 13 compares maternal body support in upright postures with BN, across a range of laid-back maternal body slopes.

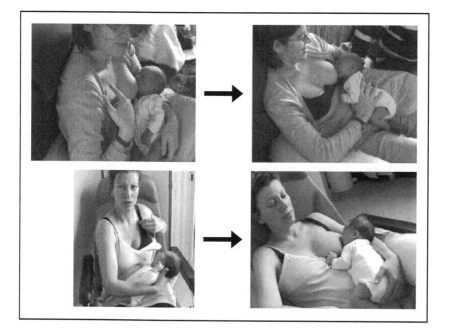

Figure 13. Maternal Body Support from Upright to BN Postures
Photos © Suzanne Colson.

Read what one student midwife wrote:

Dear Suzanne,

I am fascinated by the BN approach but I have never before put into practice your ideas. Until now! I attended a new mum on a Postnatal Visit at home who was experiencing problems with latching and sore nipples. When I arrived, she seemed a bit distressed and her baby was crying, so I suggested we try something different to what she had been shown by the Midwives. I asked her to semi-recline and popped baby on her chest, and within about 3 minutes she self-attached. The mother was totally amazed and had no pain at all on feeding. My mentor who was with me commented on how she had never seen anything like it.

Thank you for your insight.

Angie, Student Midwife (now qualified) and breastfeeding counsellor Bournemouth, England

Chapter 8

Baby Position

One of the aims of BN is to facilitate the processes of adaptation from womb to world by finding and emphasising the points of continuity from foetus to neonate that we discussed previously. These common points are inherent in the mechanisms of biological nurturing and have immediate implications for clinical support. For example, we saw in Chapter 6 that PNRs develop from 28 gestational weeks so that releasing them at birth in the breastfeeding context builds upon something familiar for both mother and baby.

Another Point of Continuity: Neonatal Lie

When lying prone in a physiological body tilt on top of the gentle maternal body slope, we observed that the baby often moves into a position similar to how he was lying in the womb (albeit head up). This point of continuity from foetus to neonate leads to further clarification of the concept of neonatal lie.

When a mother sits upright, she is taught a fixed postural system, maintaining her back at right angles to her lap; this approximate 90° angle closes her body, limiting the space available to her baby. The mother, therefore, usually holds her baby at right angles to her body. The baby inevitably lies in a transverse position across, by, or around her midriff (Figure 14).

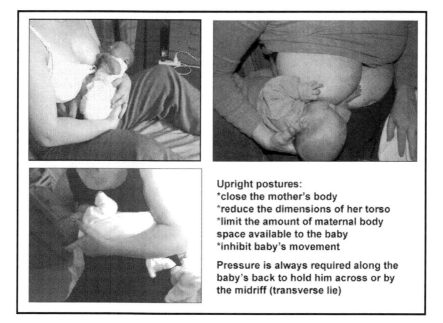

Upright postures:
*close the mother's body
*reduce the dimensions of her torso
*limit the amount of maternal body
space available to the baby
*inhibit baby's movement

Pressure is always required along the
baby's back to hold him across or by
the midriff (transverse lie)

Figure 14. Positional Effects of Upright Postures
Photo upper left © Suzanne Colson; photo upper right © Trix Simmons;
photo lower left © Tom Haven.

In contrast, as soon as a mother leans back, the dimensions of her body space increase–particularly in her midriff. The round breast now lies on an open plane. The baby modifies the lie, or direction, of his position, using the motor PNRs released by frontal positional brushing with the mother's body. The baby can now stretch out and often moves towards a lie that is up and down or obliquely on top of the mother's body (Figure 15).

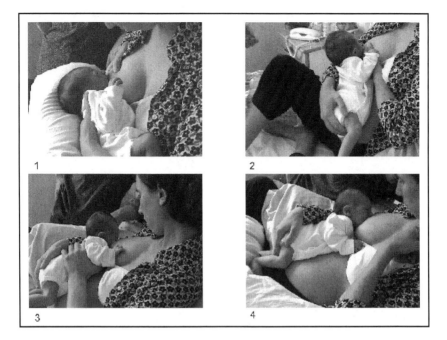

Figure 15. Positional Effects of Laid-back Postures
Photos © Suzanne Colson.

Indeed, a real advantage to BN is that babies can manoeuvre around the breast, like the hands of a clock, therefore approaching the areola from any direction. Anytime there are latching problems or flat or sore nipples, modifications to the baby's lie can be made quickly and easily by suggesting that the mother lean back. As soon as she opens her body, the baby then manoeuvres to the familiar positional direction.

Neonatal lie, therefore, is a key subcomponent of the baby's position. The term is borrowed from the obstetrical/midwifery assessments of "foetal lie" made during pregnancy. Foetal lie is formally defined as a relation between the long axis of the baby's body to the long axis of the mother's womb. The definition is easily applied to the neonatal period. Neonatal lie formally describes the relation between the long part of the baby to the long part of the mother. Like foetal lie, three positional directions can be identified: longitudinal, transverse, and oblique. If you look closely at Figure 16, you will see the different positional directions or ways to approach the breast, as well as one baby who is about to "head right". He looks like a swimmer. His head is turned away from the mid-line, the head-righting reflex will bring his head into the midline.

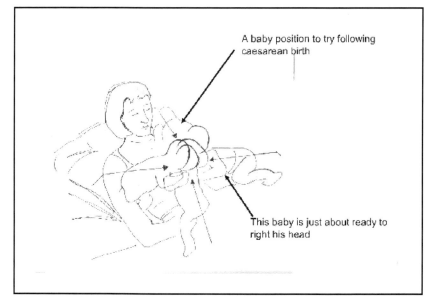

Figure 16. The Versatility of Neonatal Lie
Line drawing © Suzanne Carter.

Normally, the foetus lies longitudinally in late pregnancy, although the incidence of a transverse foetal lie is 1 in 300 to 400 at delivery (Cockburn & Drake, 1969; Wood & Forster, 2005). A transverse foetal lie, if sustained during labour, leads to a malpresentation, that is, the shoulder is usually the presenting part and a caesarean will be required.

My breastfeeding data suggest that many babies self-attach spontaneously in positions where the maternal body slope accommodates a longitudinal or oblique neonatal lie similar to the womb position. Following normal birth, the lie of the three baby holds (cradle, cross-cradle, and rugby/football) that mothers are taught to use are transverse, placing the baby in an unfamiliar lie. It is therefore not surprising that mothers must also be taught a fixed way to attach the baby onto the breast. Malpresentation or position is a frequent cause of caesarean section. When mothers have had caesarean births, the baby can approach the breast in a transverse or oblique lie, even over-the mother's shoulder. In that way, mothers do not have to worry about the baby kicking or moving against the recent wound.

Read in Figure 17 what a mother of a six-day-old baby said:

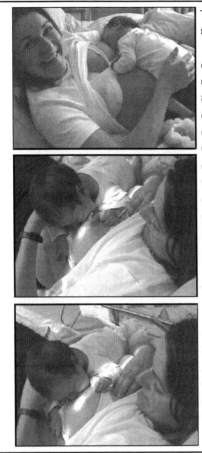

The mother of this six day old baby said:

"I get the impression that this [laid-back] position has always helped her to digest really well; when her body is like this it goes down well; she's never vomited. I have both hands free and I have no tension in my back. I had lots of contractions during feeds in the beginning and it really helped because she was like a little hot water bottle ...I feel relaxed and, she is immediately right across from the breast; there are no risks that she will damage my nipple; she takes it all in her mouth. It's much less strenuous than positions where you have to hold the baby with your arms; usually it's your arms that carry the baby whereas my baby carries herself. I was convinced that having a caesarean meant you couldn't breastfeed but the midwives put her on my tummy straight away and I was determined to make breastfeeding work.... to make up for the birth."

Figure 17.
Photos © Suzanne Colson.

Mothers with large or pendulous breasts or who are obese or dysmorphic, short arm length, for example, can use any comfortable laid-back sacral sitting posture. The baby then can be placed lying, like a suckling puppy, with his tummy hugging a part of the mother's body and the bed, instead of being completely on top of the mother (Figure 18).

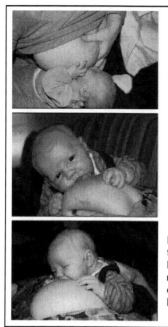

Mother sits upright clutching baby in rugby hold. She supports and compresses her breast with one hand and holds the baby's back with the other. Her hand and arm take the full weight of the baby

Mother leans back; baby approaches the breast in an oblique lie, mother gathers her breast with one hand, the other is free

Now in a transverse lie, the baby has access to the breast, in an open plane, from the side. He latches and feeds, his tummy hugs his mother's torso and bed. Mother has at least one hand but often both hands free. She can let go of the baby's lower back.

Figure 18. Storyboard: Large Breasted Mother Leans Back
Photos © Trix Simmons.

Figure 19 recounts how an assessment of neonatal lie helped a mother whose baby was in a breech presentation come to terms with her sore nipples.

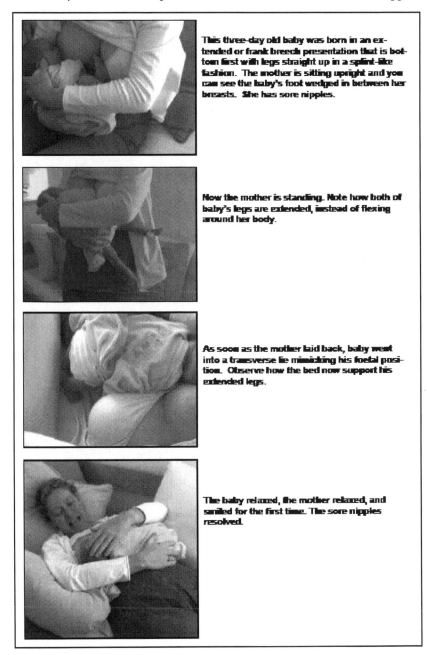

This three-day old baby was born in an extended or frank breech presentation that is bottom first with legs straight up in a splint-like fashion. The mother is sitting upright and you can see the baby's foot wedged in between her breasts. She has sore nipples.

Now the mother is standing. Note how both of baby's legs are extended, instead of flexing around her body.

As soon as the mother laid back, baby went into a transverse lie mimicking his foetal position. Observe how the bed now support his extended legs.

The baby relaxed, the mother relaxed, and smiled for the first time. The sore nipples resolved.

Figure 19. Breech Baby Story Board.
Photos © Suzanne Colson.

Lessons From Other Mammals

An understanding of the concept of neonatal lie makes us think about the positions other mammals use to feed.

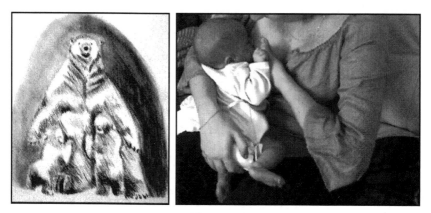

Figure 20.
Line drawing © Ken Tackett. Photo © Suzanne Colson.

Look at the pictures of a polar bear and a human mother both breastfeeding upright in Figure 20 above. We do not need a tape measure to say that the distance in inches between the sternum and the pubis of the polar bear is greater than that of the human mother. The polar bear mother does not need to hold her babies, applying pressure on their backs, necks, or heads. Verticality seems to work a treat for the polar bear, but not so well for the human mother. Comparatively, although it is possible for the human neonate to breastfeed, held vertically in front of and parallel to the mother's torso, this position looks awkward, uncomfortable for both mother and baby. Verticality looks difficult to sustain for the human mother. Unlike the polar bear, the human mother who is upright has to hold her baby, applying pressure along the baby's back. When the mother holds her baby upright, her arm pressure boxes the baby into her body, limiting neonatal locomotion. The baby is somewhat stuck in the midriff unable to move up or down. The PNR movements are either suppressed, wasted, or expressed as barriers. See how the neonate's feet and legs are in contact with thin air. Placing and stepping will not help the baby self attach in this position. The mother must control latch and milk transfer.

Now look at what happens in Figure 21 below as soon as the mother lays back: everything seems to change almost immediately.

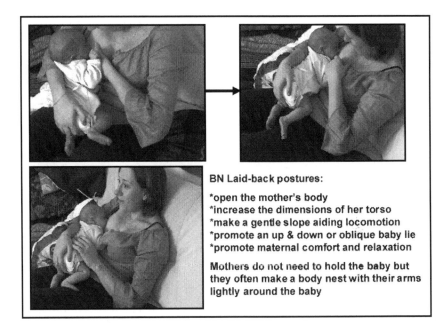

Figure 21.
Photos © Suzanne Colson.

These observations lead us to speculate: Are feeding positions species-specific? And if so, does the positive use of gravity play a central role? That topic is the subject of the next chapter.

Chapter 9

Species Specificity and Gravitational Mechanisms

All living creatures are subjected to the forces of gravity. The more upright we are, the greater the burden. From an evolutionary perspective, it makes sense that each species would have anti-gravity strategies aiding them to accomplish those activities that are necessary for survival.

In my study, laid-back mother postures enabled full-frontal breastfeeding positions, similar to those used by some of our mammalian cousins. Using gravity positively, there is an argument to suggest that these positions may be species-specific to the human neonate, as it must be recalled that the human animal is not upright until the end of the first year of life.

The Positive Use of Gravity

Certainly, the positive use of gravity was integral to the success of biological nurturing and influenced two important mechanical factors. First, gravity promoted close mother-baby body apposition. Second, gravity smoothed jerky reflex movements, promoting neonatal locomotion when the degree of maternal body slope was favourable. In turn, these factors appeared to influence the synergy between BN postures and positions. Therefore, the force of gravity played a central role in the expression of the reflexes—either as stimulants or as barriers to successful breastfeeding.

The mechanisms have to do with gravitational drag exerting pressure, which draws the baby towards the centre of the earth. When a breastfeeding mother sits upright, gravity drags the baby straight down the maternal torso towards the pillow, the mother's lap, and the floor. The baby's reflex movements, released through positional brushing, often appear jerky and uncoordinated. The more upright the mother, the greater the amplitude of those baby movements, such as hand-to-mouth and arm and leg cycling, so often associated with breast fighting or latch refusal. The greater the amplitude, the stronger the mother must grip her baby's back and neck to keep baby in place and at breast level.

In contrast, laid-back maternal sitting postures use gravity positively. The direction of the centre of the earth shifts and that same gravitational drag pulls the baby through the mother's body, maintaining close body apposition and helping to keep him in place. The amplitude of the jerky reflex movements is somewhat blunted. Mothers no longer need to hold on tightly to the baby's back, neck, or head, although mothers trying BN for the first time often apply light pressure to support the baby's head (see Figure 22).

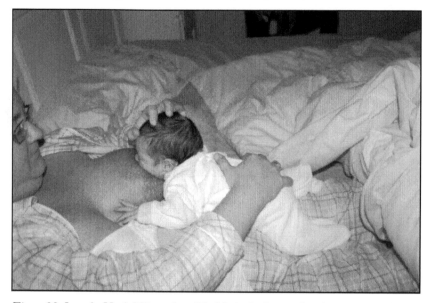

Figure 22. Janneke Hoek-Nijssen from The Netherlands uses this photo taken of her and baby, Ismee, to show mothers how to get started with biological nurturing. Photo © Johan Hoek.

Some people have asked about milk flow in BN positions, wondering how the milk can flow upward to the baby seemingly against gravity. Of course, this would not be a good position for bottle-feeding. However, we know that the breastfed baby extracts the milk aided by the milk ejection reflex. Oftentimes, the milk ejection reflex is very strong, and many babies have difficulty controlling the flow. A laid-back breastfeeding position helps with this. First, the strong flow is somewhat reduced by gravity. Second, the baby, with no pressure along his back, neck, or head, controls the feed and often comes off spontaneously, waiting for the flow to calm.

Weight is another factor that influences the force of gravitational drag. The more the baby weighs, the greater the pull of gravity. This may be one explanation why some mothers who sit upright to breastfeed develop sore nipples after the first couple of weeks.

Protecting the Frontal Region of the Body

The baby's suckling maturity and weight are just two factors that will influence the degree of maternal recline. Other factors are unrelated to physics and include the degree of privacy. The frontal region (the area from the sternum to the pubis) of the human body is an extremely sensitive area and may play an important role in close physical relationships. People may feel exposed in public situations when their frontal region is undressed or unprotected. For example, when people feel threatened or unsafe in social situations, they often send unconscious, but defensive body barrier signals that cover the frontal region of the body (Morris, 1977). Morris illustrates that when diplomats arrive in a foreign country, they take measures to conceal or protect this body area. Prior to greeting a public figure on foreign territory, a woman dignitary may reach across her body to her purse, making a temporary bar across the front torso, whereas a man may straighten his cuff links, bringing both hands in front of his body in a body cross. Both may extend one arm across the body whilst shaking hands.

This need to protect the frontal body region in public situations may be an unconscious reason motivating many mothers to sit upright to breastfeed, holding the baby across their midriff when they are out, at home with visitors, or when people take photos. In any case, once the reflexes are conditioned, the degree of body slope is less important. Furthermore, there is not one ideal degree of body slope, and when mothers are in more "public" situations, it is still possible to use gravity positively by leaning back into a comfortable sitting posture reliant upon both ischial and sacral support (see Figure 23).

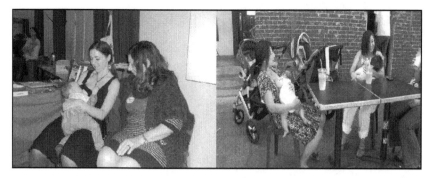

Figure 23. Biological Nurturing When Out and About

In the photo on the right, these mothers are doing BN with their babies while having coffee. Photo © Colson, Frantz, and Makelin: Biological Nurturing for Mothers DVD. *In the photo on the left, Elaine Scully from London is sitting next to me after a public conference. Read below how she now shares BN positions with other mothers. Photo © Marion Jones.*

Dear Suzanne,

I've been meaning to contact you, to say thank you for your talk at the Enrichment Day. A few weeks after, I met a new mum at our café who was already sitting in the Biological Nurturing position with her son asleep on her, as she told me their history and how much of a struggle feeding is. I used a doll to show how from where she is, she could latch her baby on, and then when he woke up she tried it.

Mum exclaimed with joy! She wanted to know why no one else had ever told her about this, as when her baby had struggled in the start, the hospital had told her to use a very mechanical "holding breast and baby's head and forcing together" method. He fed like a dream afterwards.

And from there I've gone on to promoting it to many mothers, with babies and antenatally. I knew of BN before, but after the enrichment day I felt far better equipped to suggest it to others.

Parallel Angles on Birth and Breastfeeding

We have had some scientific evidence demonstrating how gravity affects labour and birth for over a quarter of a century. There is an interesting parallel to be made between BN and the positional changes for birth proposed in the

1980s. Freedom of position is often restricted during labour. During active management, for example, the foetal heart rate must be assessed following surgical rupture of the membranes. Mothers usually sit semi-reclined in bed and are strapped to a monitor.

A prime index of progress in labour is the descent of the foetal head. Optimally, with each contraction, pressure is applied evenly down the foetal axis, reaching the presenting part (usually the vertex of the flexed foetal head). This pressure aids cervical dilatation. An upright or all fours position works with gravity, promoting foetal descent and opening the cervix. When mothers are recumbent, semi-recumbent, or sitting on the bed, labour contractions may be less effective, as they work against gravity. During labour, these laid-back maternal positions close the pelvis, exerting constant sacral pressure, making the ischial-sacral and the coccyx joints immobile and, as a result, often delay the descent of the foetal head.

Nevertheless, obstetricians and midwives traditionally encouraged mothers to give birth lying on their sides, in a Semi-Fowlers position, or with their feet in stirrups in a lithotomy position. American midwife Ina May Gaskin (1977), anthropologist Sheila Kitzinger (1972), childbirth educator Janet Balaskas (1983), and French obstetrician Michel Odent (1984) were some of the first to suggest that being upright during labour and birth has mechanical advantages, using gravity positively. Although freedom of position during labour and birth immediately resonated with many mothers, many health professionals remained unconvinced, leading to heated debate. Today in the UK, it is recognised that the positive use of gravity reduces the need for pharmaceutical pain relief and helps to keep birth "normal".

Likewise the "laid-back" breastfeeding postures, the most important component of biological nurturing, also challenge our beliefs about the best position to use when breastfeeding, sometimes creating heated discussion. Many mothers immediately embraced the concept, but a number of health practitioners remain sceptical.

In both instances, the postures suggested for centuries as "correct" to achieve a reproductive outcome did not take into account gravitational forces. There is a certain irony in that our assumptions about the correct positions for birth work for breastfeeding and those for breastfeeding work for birth. Our beliefs and convictions have been turned on their heads–by gravity!

We next turn our attention to the final component of biological nurturing: the impact of mother and baby behavioural states.

Chapter 10

Baby and Mother Behavioural States

Neonatal Behavioural State: Definitions and Results

Neonatal behavioural state has been defined as a group of physiological and motor characteristics that occur together, indicating levels of arousal; body, eye, and facial movements are observed, along with heart rate and breathing patterns (Brazelton & Nugent, 1995, Prechtl, 1974, 1977; Wolff, 1959, 1966). For my research, I borrowed definitions from the observable variables used by Wolff (1987), Brazelton and Nugent (1995, 1999), and enhanced by Blackburn (2003) and Biancuzzo (1999).

My research definitions included the six neonatal behavioural states defined by Brazelton and Nugent (1995). In addition, and importantly, I identified three sleep and three awake states, whereas traditionally, a drowsy state (in between asleep and awake) is usually called an awake state. The three sleep states were deep, light, and drowsy. The three awake states were active/quiet alert, fussy (crying for less than 1 minute), and crying (Figure 24).

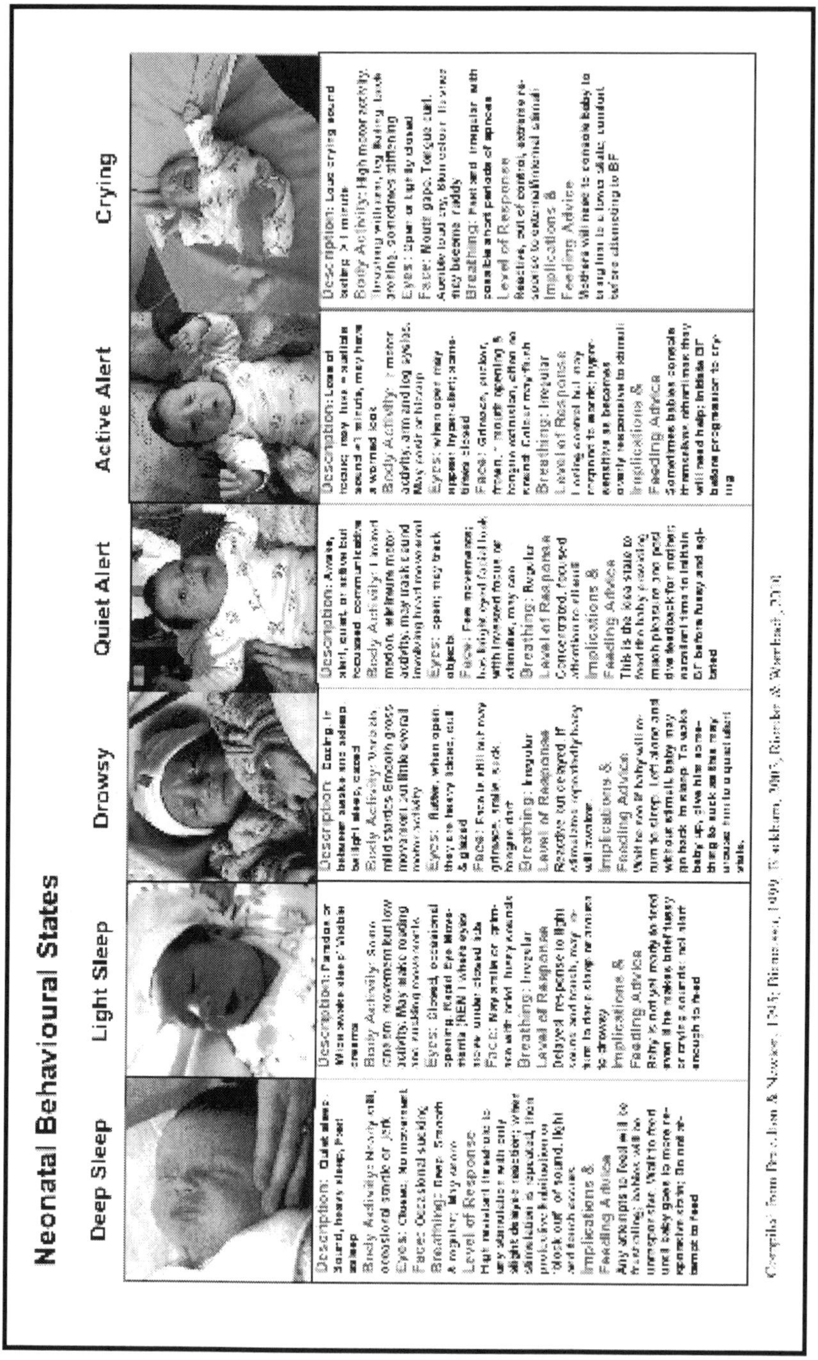

Figure 24. Neonatal Behavioural States

Photos © Suzanne Colson. Text compiled from Brazelton & Newton, 1995; Biancusso, 1999; Blackburn, 2003, Riordan & Wambach, 2010.

The research episodes commenced when mothers picked their babies up with feeding intention. The results demonstrated that two PNRs were not observed in the sleep states, leg cycling and crawling. The others were observed in both sleep and awake states, with no association between neonatal behavioural state and the number of reflexes observed either at latch or at milk transfer.

Traditionally, mothers have been encouraged to feed their babies in awake states, with the quiet alert state being optimal (Biancuzzo, 1999; Blackburn, 2003; Brazelton & Nugent, 1995; Koehn & Riordan, 2010; Prechtl, 1977). In my study, the babies in both the bottle- and breastfeeding groups latched on and fed in sleep states. However, consistent with paediatric findings, the strength of PNR response was somewhat diminished.

Behavioural State Mechanisms

If you were to ask 100 mothers how they know their baby needs to feed, it is likely that they would all say it is because the baby cries. This probably happens because people think that babies should feed in awake states. However, my results suggest that variations from light sleep to quiet alert states are compatible with breastfeeding, whereas fussy and crying states often complicate everything, making it impossible for some babies to latch. Crying is accepted culturally as the normal verbal way for a baby to indicate hunger. However, from a human-needs perspective, crying for food indicates that your most basic needs are not being met. Imagine if adults had to burst into tears to indicate they were ready for dinner every evening!

The BN value system places great importance upon keeping the baby in his natural habitat. This, of course, is the mother's body, even when the baby is asleep. During sleep, babies cue in various ways, and when mothers hold their babies, they respond sooner, recognising the cues. The results of my study suggest that BN positional interactions released PNRs as stimulants, even when the baby was observed to be in sleep states. This evidence challenges the well-documented belief that "a sleeping baby will not feed and a hungry baby will not sleep". This also calls into question the necessity of any baby, in our industrialised world, having to cry for a feed.

People often ask, "Why would anyone hold a sleeping baby?" There are two main reasons. Deep sleep is anabolic, promoting growth and development. Having three to four full sleep cycles during a nap is restorative. When you BN a sleeping baby, you protect the integrity of the sleep cycle and increase the opportunity to have repeated sleep cycles. This happens because the maternal body nest is a familiar place; mothers spontaneously reduce any effects from environmental disturbances.

Second and importantly, during the sleep cycle, babies often latch on and breastfeed. This happens because, just as in awake states, the body brushing releases PNR latching behaviours.

Let us examine some general information and evidence explaining how babies' sleep patterns progress from foetus to neonate.

General Information

Active/light sleep has been termed "wide-awake sleep" and is associated with learning. This is because brain activity is similar to brain waves in awake states. Babies, like adults, process information which is entered into memory. Sleep patterns change as the central nervous system develops: motor activity occurs during sleep and awake states in both the foetus and the neonate (Blackburn, 2003).

Foetal Life

Sleep-wake behavioural states, with organised patterns of rest and activity cycles, develop at approximately 32 gestational weeks. These states are determined by heart rate, REM (rapid eye movements), and body movements. Active/light sleep, characterised by REM (rapid eye movements), develops from 28 to 30 gestational weeks, whereas quiet/deep sleep develops at approximately 36 gestational weeks. The foetal state cycle consists of changes from REM (light) sleep to awake states, and lasts about 40 minutes (Blackburn, 2003; Brazelton & Nugent, 1995; Nijhuis, Prechtl, Martin, & Botts, 1982).

Neonatal Life

At birth, the newborn sleeps for up to 18 hours a day, but neonatal sleep is neither diurnal nor does it follow a light/dark pattern. The brand-newborn sleep cycle lasts approximately the same amount of time as the foetal cycle (from 20 to 50 minutes). This is approximately half the length of the adult sleep cycle (90 minutes). As neonatal sleep function matures, there is an increase in the duration of deep sleep, and a decrease in periods of light REM or active sleep, with a greater number of full sleep cycles occurring consecutively. This lengthens nap times and extends the duration of nighttime sleep (Blackburn, 2003; Brazelton & Nugent, 1995; Wolff, 1959). Taken together, this evidence suggests that increased sleep duration is a natural part of growth and development, not reliant on method of feeding or resulting from sleep training techniques.

Neurological Assessment

The third postnatal day is selected as optimal for evaluating neonatal neurobehaviours using the Brazelton Neonatal Behavioral Assessment Scale (NBAS) (Brazelton & Nugent, 1995). This may be because the baby has completed an initial postnatal adaptation, stabilising physiological processes. If a baby maintains an active alert state for 30 seconds during this third-day evaluation, he obtains a high score. Newborn babies change state so rapidly that during the time it takes to carry out the NBAS evaluation (15-20 minutes), the baby can change state up to 24 times (Brazelton & Nugent, 1995; Prechtl, 1977).

Integrating Facts from Sleep Research into Breastfeeding Support Practices

Because sleep states develop in the womb, there is a strong argument suggesting that mothers already know a lot about their baby's sleep. However, many new parents appear bewildered, saying that their baby certainly does not sleep three-quarters of his day! They expect their newborn to "sleep like a baby", yet this portrait is not always an accurate representation of their lived reality. Mothers often say that each time they put the baby down, instead of settling, he wakes up. This is not really surprising, and there are several biological explanations.

Change in Normal Habitat

We must remember that the baby has been held in the womb for nine months. Most babies remain asleep in a mother's arms or on her body, but as soon as baby is placed in cot or cradle, he awakens. So this is not a sleep problem per se.

Unfortunately, when this happens, instead of understanding that continuity of normal "habitat" has been disturbed, mothers often think that they have not got enough milk and that is why the baby is not settled. Health professionals believe that being "settled" and sleeping after a feed is an indicator of good milk transfer and satiety. Yet to my knowledge, there is no research data supporting this argument. Indeed, it sometimes works the opposite way: the "good baby" spending hours asleep in the cot may fail to thrive. If latching behaviours are released by positional interactions, as my data strongly suggest, then being settled in a cot is not a part of the equation.

Being settled may be a flawed index of early neonatal well-being. Another perspective suggests that it is not normal for anyone to feel "settled" when arriving in a new place, let alone a newborn baby whose every system is immature. Right after birth, being settled is not the aim. The aim is to make a successful transition from foetus to neonate. Babies who cry when placed in the cot after a feed are cueing. The crying behaviour rarely means that the mother has not got enough milk. The baby usually stops crying as soon as his mother picks him up. The crying cues, therefore, only mean that the newborn baby is not in the right place.

Baby's Short Sleep Cycle

As we have seen, babies change state very quickly, even when they are in the right place. Brazelton and Nugent (1995) suggest that behavioural state control is a window into the baby's neural-organisation and social and interactive maturity. Yet on the third postnatal day (i.e., the best time to carry out an evaluation), few babies sustain a quiet alert state for very long. As we discussed in Chapter 6, the "quality" of being alert is measured by the amount of time during which the baby has focused attention on a stimulus without turning away to return to either a sleep state or a hyper-alert fussy state (Brazelton & Nugent, 1995). The ease of state transition, sometimes termed state modulation, is also assessed as part of the NBAS. Babies score well when there are smooth transitions and alert periods are prolonged, lasting for 30 seconds or more. The duration of the time spent in a quiet alert state helps to assess how the baby responds and controls his response to environmental stimuli, although many newborns are quickly overwhelmed (Brazelton & Nugent, 1995).

Many mothers are left feeling confused by the quality and quantity of sleep necessary to promote their baby's well-being. Few health professionals, however, routinely discuss neonatal behavioural states, the rapid state changes, and the resulting abrupt and fluctuating sleep patterns. Doing BN with the sleeping baby during the first postnatal weeks is a way for mothers to assess their baby's individual sleep patterns. Mothers protect baby's sleep states, temperature, and breathing all at the same time. In that way, they get to know their baby's rhythms and needs more quickly. Because the neonatal sleep cycle is so short and the capacity for deep sleep so immature, many babies do not sleep well on their own. In the first weeks, doing BN may help to develop smooth transitions and keep babies in deep sleep longer.

Babies who are held and carried also cry less, conserving both maternal and neonatal energy, as well as increasing the maternal enjoyment that should go hand-in-hand with having a new baby. Once breastfeeding feels established, some mothers will opt to continue to carry the baby a lot, using a sling. Many health professionals tell mothers that putting a baby down, back to sleep in a cot, is the only acceptable way to support sleep. It has been over 40 years since Montagu (1971) suggested that a period of external gestation is beneficial for mothers and babies! Is it not time for health professionals to share this message with mothers?

Counterpoint: What About the State of the Mother?

We were also able to identify maternal behavioural states and, interestingly, these appeared to be related to the mother's posture. As soon as mothers laid back, they looked and acted differently. They seemed to change state: going from thinking, concentrating, or worrying to a state of relaxation. This led them to focus upon their baby. It was unclear whether relaxation was the result, or the releaser, of this change. For a mother who had breastfeeding problems, it was like she discovered her baby for the first time. For all the mothers, the gentle body slope supported natural gazing behaviours. They could look at their baby without craning their necks. In turn, simply looking at the baby appeared to release a cascade of innate maternal behaviours. I interpreted this phenomenon as likely being associated with high levels of oxytocin pulsatility.

The Role of Oxytocin

Oxytocin, a peptide hormone, is well known for its contraction and ejection effects. Produced in the hypothalamus and stored in the posterior pituitary gland, oxytocin is not released in a steady stream, but rather in pulses, and high peaks of pulsatility are associated with orgasm, ejaculation, foetus ejection, and milk release (Odent, 1987; Uvnäs-Moberg, 2003). The contraction/ejection effects are often termed mechanical or peripheral because they can be caused to occur artificially through the intravenous infusion of synthetic oxytocin (trademarked syntocinon or pitocin). The synthetic form is often used to contract the uterus to augment labour or is mixed with ergometrine to control postpartum bleeding. The synthetic molecule is too large to cross the blood-brain barrier and, therefore, pitocin, or syntocinon, remains peripheral, achieving good contraction and ejection effect. However, it is noteworthy that this does not impact maternal emotional state (McNabb, 1997b; Uvnäs-Moberg, 2003).

There is an increasing body of good quality research evidence suggesting that oxytocin also has central, behavioural effects, which only occur when it is released into the blood stream directly by the brain; the effects of which, many studies have suggested, promote social, sexual, and maternal behaviours (Herbert, 1994; Pedersen, 1992; Uvnäs-Moberg, 2003). That is why so many people now call oxytocin the "love or cuddle hormone".

It is well known that a hospital or home environment during labour conducive to high oxytocin pulsatility is associated with normal vaginal birth without any need for intervention. However, the potential effects of the maintenance of high maternal concentrations into the early postnatal weeks are less well known. Results from research carried out by Uvnäs-Moberg and her team from Sweden suggest that this may be important. For example:

- Maternal oxytocin concentrations are higher immediately following birth than at any time during labour (Uvnäs-Moberg, 1989).

- Higher maternal oxytocin pulsatility on the second postnatal day is associated with increased breastfeeding duration at six weeks (Nissen et al., 1996).

Oxytocin has an anti-stress effect. Each suckling episode is followed by a decrease in blood pressure, and breastfeeding mothers are calmer. This correlates with oxytocin concentrations (Uvnäs-Moberg, 1997; 1998).

Furthermore, observations by midwives, like Ina May Gaskin (1977), and obstetricians, like Michel Odent (1992; 1999; 2004), have described some physical and behavioural characteristics of people who appear to be under the influence of oxytocin. These include eyes closed or half-closed, mouth open or half smile, and facial or body flush. Odent (1999) suggests that women giving birth appear to be completely unaware of their surroundings, disconnected from the world–"on another planet." However, Kendall-Tackett (2010) suggests that health professionals need to recognise the difference between a mother who is transported by events and one who is in a dissociative state because of prior or current psychological trauma.

Observations of mothers who are transported by events are supported by some research evidence suggesting that oxytocin induces states of euphoria and forgetfulness (Pedersen, 1992). Marsha Walker (2002) suggests that uterine contractions, sometimes called after pains experienced during breastfeeding, are also indicators of successful milk transfer, although this kind of observation only reflects the mechanical effects of high oxytocin concentrations. Building upon Walker's observations, close, but discrete, observations of the mothers in my study revealed erect nipples that could also be interpreted as mechanical indicators. Increased thirst is yet another index that research suggests is associated with high oxytocin pulsatility, and it is well known that breastfeeding mothers increase their fluid intake (Bentley, 1998).

Just as clusters of features define neonatal behaviour states, theoretically, it is possible that these observations could be viewed as part of a hormonal profile supporting lactation. I introduced new terminology to describe these emerging behavioural patterns suggestive of high maternal oxytocin pulsatility. Instead of saying a "maternal behavioural state indicative of high oxytocin pulsatility", I used an umbrella term, *hormonal complexion*, to indicate this or any group of physical and behavioural features appearing to occur regularly and together, suggestive of high levels of a hormone.

Within the expert group that supported the PhD work, we continue to discuss theories that might underpin these surprising findings. Today, "hormonal complexion" is being developed as a theoretical construct. It is not unusual to associate colours with emotions and physical states of being: green with envy, red with anger or heat or a flush of excitement, and blue with melancholy. Similarly stress, frustration, fear, and fight-and-flight behaviours (especially where reaction is inhibited) can be observed as biochemical responses in people's facial expressions suggesting, for example, a cortisol or an adrenalin complexion.

The theory here suggests that an oxytocic complexion goes hand-in-hand with the expression of the innate maternal behaviours observed, such as nesting, greeting, olfactory, transportation, grooming, body placing, gaze, and imitation. These findings exceed the scope and purpose of this book. Nevertheless, compelling video data suggest that human mothers have a species-specific innate behavioural capacity to breastfeed (Figure 25).

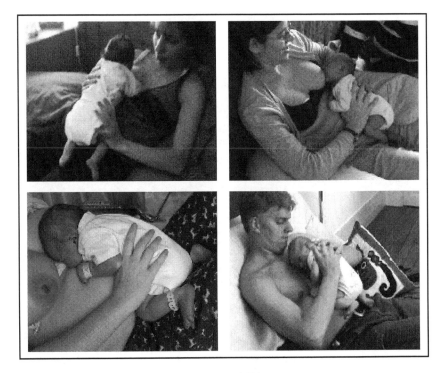

Figure 25. Body Placing
Photos © Suzanne Colson.

This figure illustrates one such universal behaviour observed across the sample. When mothers and fathers are in positions of relaxation, with their babies on top of their bodies, variations of the position called ventral suspension can be observed. I termed this spontaneous response "body placing".

Let us recall that ventral suspension concerns holding the baby around the thorax and is one of three positions used by paediatricians to release PNRs, like placing, walking, and stepping. Interestingly, as soon as anyone does BN, they appear to place the baby up their bodies, even if there is no breastfeeding intent (like the father pictured above). Universal behaviour is a characteristic of an instinct, defined as an inborn or unlearned action, common to the species, having a fixed behavioural pattern without conscious intent (Brown, 1993; McFarland, 2006). The releaser of this behaviour appeared to be full frontal contact, independent of the state of dress.

Observe the intimate baby focus. We know that even looking at a photo of a baby can release or increase oxytocin pulsatility, and this is one reason why I associated this phenomenon with a hormonal complexion conducive to breastfeeding. The hormonal theory supporting these observations is summarised below (see textbox).

Theory for Maternal Hormonal Complexion

(Colson & Greenfield, 2006)

We have said previously that changing from upright to laid-back postures often induces a state of relaxation and what we have described as an oxytocic maternal complexion. Breastfeeding mothers were observed to alter their behaviours during episodes of BN. These changes seemed to coincide with a physical shift from reliance upon ischial sitting to sacral sitting. The before/after BN observations from the videotapes were so striking that we started thinking about possible explanations, and a physiological mechanism for these behavioural changes slowly emerged. As mothers changed from upright to laid-back postures, the movements of sacral nutation and counter-nutation (see Figure 9) occurred.

Physiologically, this movement, well recognised by cranial osteopaths, could travel up the spinal column to release a burst of oxytocin, which we can recall is stored in the posterior pituitary gland. Therefore, it is possible that central release of oxytocin could be influenced by complex systems of sacral/occipital miming actions. Simply put, through flexion of the sacrum, a mother could, theoretically, be stimulating her pituitary gland.

We acknowledge that the potential mechanism proposed for this phenomenon is purely speculative, as no blood samples to measure maternal oxytocin concentrations were taken to give any physiological credence to these interpretations. However, these compelling visual data build upon the increasing amount of well-designed research carried out by Kerstin Uvnäs-Moberg and her colleagues in Sweden, examining oxytocin and its behavioural effects, where blood samples were taken. Biological nurturing may be an intervention increasing oxytocin pulsatility as a bridging hormone from pregnancy to lactation. Further research is clearly required.

Chapter 11

How Does Biological Nurturing Compare with Skin-to-Skin Contact?

We have just reviewed what is known about the mechanisms of biological nurturing. Some would argue that these are complex and difficult to understand. However, the intervention itself is quick and easy to do. It is similar to encouraging mothers to hold their babies in skin-to-skin contact. However, there are some key differences.

Skin-to-skin is now promoted as being crucial to breastfeeding initiation, with mothers advised to do it from birth until the baby has his first feed, and to continue during the first postnatal days. We know there are different degrees of skin-to-skin, and there may be different definitions. What is rarely discussed is that mothers are sometimes uncomfortable with prolonged bare skin contact, especially after the first postnatal hours. The aim of this chapter is to clarify important differences between BN and skin-to-skin contact and examine aspects of the evidence base.

A Brief History of Skin-to-Skin Contact

When we trace the history of skin-to-skin, we can see it is sometimes called Kangaroo Mother Care (KMC) and was originally conceived as life support for preterm infants in countries in the developing world (Rey & Martinez, 1983). I have vivid memories of my first professional contact with KMC. In 1984, I was working as a lactation consultant at Pithiviers State Hospital in France, where I held weekly breastfeeding meetings. Pregnant and new mothers came along for informal discussions about birth, breastfeeding, and life with a new baby. One evening, a healthy but moderately preterm baby was born following a normal vaginal birth in the *salle sauvage*, the home-like maternity environment that Michel Odent and his team designed with the help of some of the parents who gave birth there.

The preterm baby, born the night before my meeting, appeared healthy, was breathing air, and was stable. Odent, chief of staff at the time, did a very innovative thing. He decided not to transfer the baby to the tertiary unit in Orleans. The baby was really tiny, perfect, and beautiful, and I still remember the red bathrobe the mother wore to keep her baby in place, prone and upright, in skin-to-skin contact between her breasts. She looked so happy and, of course, she wanted to breastfeed. So she attended our group discussion with her baby who slept and breastfed the whole time. The baby was exclusively breastfed from birth, and the mother carried on breastfeeding. This was not really surprising, as most of the mothers who came to Pithiviers had normal births and breastfed. The caesarean rate at the time was 7%. These were such exciting times. The late Dominique Acolet was the official paediatrician at Pithiviers, and he left shortly after that for Central America to study more about KMC. I left shortly thereafter, a fervent promoter of skin-to-skin contact, to do my midwifery training.

Kangaroo Care

Imported to industrialised countries by such pioneers as Anderson, Luddington-Hoe, and Bergman, skin-to-skin contact from birth is now encouraged for all neonates—not just preterm babies. Defined as placing the naked, nappy-clad newborn baby prone on the mother's bare chest, Anderson and colleagues (2004) suggest that skin-to-skin contact provides a mammalian-specific "habitat". This promotes olfactory stimulation and innate feeding behaviours, enabling babies to find the breast and latch spontaneously.

This time frame could represent a sensitive period for priming mothers and infants to develop a synchronous, reciprocal interaction pattern provided they are together in intimate contact (Moore & Anderson, 2005, p. 488).

Whilst these points concerning place and time are agreed, the biological nurturing argument suggests that innate behaviours are released anytime mothers and babies bodies are in full frontal contact, even when mothers and babies are lightly dressed. Therefore, there is a shift in emphasis. What is important in BN is to keep mothers and babies comfortable and together, in close frontal contact, maintaining the species-specific habitat. In that way, the mother's body provides continuity from foetus to neonate. Even in conditions where mothers and babies are lightly dressed, if babies are not swaddled, there is still ample opportunity for intimate tactile and sensory stimulation. Furthermore, the notion that skin-to-skin contact is a mammalian strategy does not appear entirely accurate when we examine positions used by other animals. For example, cows, horses, and sheep stand to feed with minimal maternal contact, and abdominal feeders, such as puppies, kittens, hamsters, pigs, mice, and rats nurse with their tummies hugging the ground. This is not skin-to-skin contact.

My Experience

My own experience of this sensitive time period is mixed: my first baby was born in 1973 by forceps following a long and difficult labour. We were separated at birth for about 24 hours, but thereafter he hardly left my arms. I breastfed exclusively for over six months, and we continued into toddlerhood when he self-weaned. Interestingly, research findings (Widstrom et al., 1987) suggest that routine mother-baby separation for interventions, such as gastric suctioning, weighing, measuring, and dressing, can disrupt early innate behavioural patterns having a negative impact upon breastfeeding duration.

Odent (1977) concurs, viewing this time as a critically sensitive period when mothers and babies, awake and alert, share a reciprocal and unique hormonal state, with high oxytocic (OT) pulsatility priming the early expression of the rooting reflex. Findings from more recent research carried out by Bystova and her colleagues (2007) suggest that infants separated from their mothers for 120 minutes after birth, and then rooming in, had similar fourth-day breastfeeding outcomes as those babies with no postpartum separation held in skin-to-skin contact or lightly dressed contact.

During my second pregnancy, I was well into my La Leche League leader training and determined to keep my baby with me after the birth. The Klaus and Kennel book (1976) about bonding arrived in France during the last month of my pregnancy. This book boosted my confidence, and I negotiated with the hospital staff insisting upon minimal separation. With great delight, I held my brand newborn daughter immediately following her birth. I have fond personal memories of this time of skin-to-skin contact. After that, we remained alone in the recovery room for several hours. Again, I insisted upon holding her, although she had been measured and weighed and dressed in a little hospital gown.

As she was my second breastfed baby, I remember being surprised that she spent about an hour just licking my nipple before she latched. Hospital midwives frowned upon my close baby cuddling, telling me to put her in the cot and threatening nasty predictions about long-term effects of too much baby holding. Nevertheless, I spent long hours throughout the hospital stay holding and suckling my baby. We were both lightly dressed and, although I could not recall if I had used BN postures myself, photos taken at the time revealed that I often breastfed in laid-back sitting postures.

With my third baby, despite returning to the same hospital, I was only "allowed" to hold him for a few minutes after the birth. Nevertheless, as soon as I arrived in my postnatal room, I held my newborn for long periods of time, although this was not in skin-to-skin contact. I breastfed my second and third babies exclusively for around six months, and both weaned sometime between the ages of three and four.

Why Skin-To-Skin Is Not a Component of Biological Nurturing

Some may wonder why skin-to-skin contact is missing from the list of BN components set out in the previous chapters when research from all over the world demonstrates striking benefits. There are many reasons, and these are integral to my personal and clinical practice, as well as to my research findings and theories.

For example, as part of the PhD research protocol, all mothers recruited were informed of the benefits of skin-to-skin, but it was neither imposed nor discouraged. As per research procedures, the camera started to roll as soon as I arrived, filming mothers naturalistically without researcher input. It was pre-agreed that mothers would remove clothing covering the baby's legs and feet, so the camera could capture foot reflexes. I had a small portable heater with me at all times in case the room was cold. Interestingly, no mother took off more baby clothes than was necessary, although two mothers took off their own clothes because they did not want to get them wet through leaked milk.

During the videotaped feeding session, only two mothers in my study spontaneously held their babies in skin-to-skin contact: one who specifically requested to try out what she saw on the *Delivery Self Attachment* film that was shown to all the mothers recruited during pregnancy. The other gave birth at home to a baby born at 37 gestational weeks. Her midwife suggested that she remain in skin-to-skin contact as much as possible with the baby.

All research participants completed a postnatal questionnaire at around six postnatal weeks where I asked, as part of the descriptive characteristics, if they ever breastfed their babies in skin-to-skin contact. I soon discovered that there are variations in the definition. Mothers often said they held their baby skin-to-skin, and then showed me pictures where one or both were lightly dressed. Look at Figure 26. Which mothers are in skin-to-skin contact?

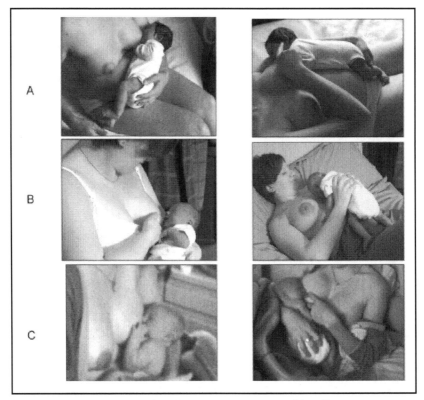

Figure 26. Mothers' Interpretation of Skin-to-Skin Contact
Photos © Suzanne Colson.

Let us also recall that at six postnatal weeks, all 40 mothers in the study, whether they practised skin-to-skin contact or not, were breastfeeding (87.5% exclusively). Time and again, variables other than skin-to-skin were observed to release PNRs and other innate behaviours as feeding stimulants. Results from 38 videotapes, where breastfeeding mothers and babies are lightly dressed, clearly indicate that positions are the key variables. For example, baby's feet tops brushed up against the maternal thigh, releasing the placing reflex aiding latch. Once latched, foot brushing along the lateral side often released a Babinski reflex. This innate toe fan expanded the baby's foot width and, like the web of a duck's foot, appeared to help the baby remain *in situ* during milk transfer.

Skin-To-Skin in an Upright Position

Photos in the bottom row of Figure 26 show the only mother filmed in a true definition for skin-to-skin contact according to the literature. She had a home birth and had been holding the baby in skin-to-skin contact since birth. When I arrived, both mother and baby were healthy, rosy, and beautiful. The mother was laid-back and comfortable, suckling her two-day-old baby, who was asleep on top of her body in her bed. However, as soon as the baby started rooting, she sat bolt upright to breastfeed as she had been taught to do with her previous baby. Although the baby latched on beautifully, the mother winced in pain as she had already developed sore nipples using this upright posture. Her experience suggests that skin-to-skin contact per se is not protective against sore nipples. During the filming, it was easy to encourage the mother to remain semi-reclined instead of being upright at latch, and the pain resolved.

It is important to highlight that when mothers breastfeed sitting upright in skin-to-skin contact, there is still the potential for the friction from positional brushing to release PNRs as barriers to latch. Upright postures, even in skin-to-skin contact, may also contribute to sore nipples through gravitational drag. Taken together, these important observations suggest that BN research, which initially built upon skin-to-skin contact, can now inform our understanding of optimal positions to use during skin-to-skin contact.

Skin-To-Skin in the First Hours

I would suggest that it makes sense to encourage all mothers to have *bare* skin-on-skin contact during the first postnatal hours because getting dressed at that time is an intervention. Research clearly demonstrates that for healthy women, one labour intervention is the first of a cascade of interventions that increases morbidity (Tew, 1995; Wagner, 2006). Likewise, Anderson, Chiu, Morrison, Burkhammer, and Ludington-Hoe (2004) highlight that "breastfeeding attempts" (p. 40) are frequently interrupted for interventions, such as genetic or auditory screening, normal paediatric examination, circumcision, hepatitis B vaccination, and photography. There is a strong argument suggesting that none of these interventions is more important than getting started with breastfeeding! An important goal for health professionals is to reduce intervention. In reproductive events, we can say with a degree of certainty that intervention will likely disrupt normality.

As night follows day, skin-to skin-contact follows on from normal birth and can easily be carried out in any birthing context: in bed following a home birth, in the delivery room following normal hospital birth, or in recovery following caesarean section. For reasons beyond comprehension, health care managers often suggest that reducing intervention will have a negative budgetary effect (Anderson et al., 2004). In fact, it is just the opposite. We have known since the early 1990s that continuity of carer is associated with better outcomes and is cost effective. I have recovered mothers having had caesarean section in skin-to-skin contact in the same bed with their babies; it is easier to recover two people, mother and baby, through concrete observations of vital signs (temperature, colour, pulse, blood pressure, and respirations), when they are together in the same bed.

Some Cautions

When we promote skin-to-skin contact immediately following birth, however, we must be aware of the effects of gravity upon both the mother's posture and the baby's position. Right after birth, mothers are often portrayed in bare skin contact lying flat on their backs with the baby lying prone and flat on top of their bodies. We need to consider these skin-to-skin positions with careful attention, as both may be disadvantageous.

Maternal Flat-Lying

Mothers are advised not to sleep flat on their backs during the last trimester of pregnancy. Midwives and doctors avoid carrying out antenatal assessments when mothers are in this position. This is because when a pregnant mother lies flat, the weight of her uterus can compress the greater blood vessels and compromise maternal blood circulation, lowering her blood pressure and reducing oxygen supply to her and her baby. Right after birth, although the uterus no longer contains the baby, it is still quite large (usually level with the mother's navel) and heavy, weighing approximately a kilo (2.2 pounds).

Odent (1992) suggests that flat-lying after birth is not a spontaneous physiological posture. His observations, spanning more than 15,000 births, suggest that following a birth without intervention, mothers who are not advised, allowed, or instructed to use a specific posture, do not lie flat on their backs. Instead following a birth using gravity positively, mothers usually greet their babies spontaneously remaining upright to deliver the placenta. Verticality continues to make positive use of gravitational forces. On the other hand, maternal flat-lying after birth, with the baby on top, increases the potential for vena cava compression, limiting the flow through this large blood vessel returning deoxygenated blood to the heart. Theoretically, the maternal flat-lying posture also increases the risk for a retained placenta.

Other reasons to avoid maternal flat-lying concern well-being. My research observations replicate what Klaus and Kennel (1976) term "the en-face position...defined as the position in which the mother's face is rotated so that her eyes and those of the infant meet fully in the same vertical plane of rotation" (p. 56). My data suggest that whatever the posture used to breastfeed, mothers gaze at their babies. When mothers are flat on their backs, even though their upper back, head, and shoulders are supported, they cannot take "the en-face position" without craning their necks upward, against gravity, and forward. Similarly, they crank their necks downward when they sit upright.

Skin-to-skin contact has no bearing upon this positional phenomenon, as can be observed in Figures 27 and 28.

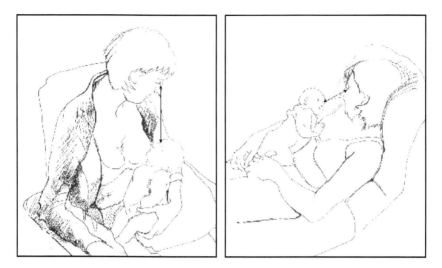

Figure 27. Postural Effects on Baby Gazing
Line drawings © Suzanne Carter.

The final reason to avoid a completely flat maternal posture concerns maternal enjoyment and control. Mothers who are flat on their backs right after birth do not look in control of events. Instead of actively initiating breastfeeding, the baby is placed by someone else on the mother's abdomen or chest, health professionals either place the mother's hand on her baby or suggest that she does not touch her baby, but wait and see what the baby will do. This kind of practice can encourage a "learned helplessness". The mother does not dare initiate, but rather looks to others for guidance. In this kind of environment, mothers often appear stressed, illustrating a cortisol hormonal complexion.

A popular video clip filmed in India shown on YouTube illustrates a mother surrounded by many people talking around her and showing her what to do (UNICEF India, 2007). Interestingly, this mother lies flat on her back, opening her body to a maximum of 180°. The baby is in a full BN position, but the mother is not. Positional brushing releases the PNRs responsible for the baby's breast crawl, just as positional friction released the innate baby reflexes, aiding latching and suckling behaviours in my research. Nevertheless, even though the baby latches in the video clip, the mother looks helpless, with people doing everything for her.

Maternal flat-lying, with or without skin-to-skin contact, is not a BN posture, although for my research, it was defined as "partial BN" because the position is optimal for the release of the baby reflexes. A biological nurturing posture is always a laid-back sitting posture; the body slope is individual to the degree of recline that facilitates relaxed mother-baby gazing, grooming, and spontaneous or innate maternal/infant breastfeeding behaviours (see Figure 28).

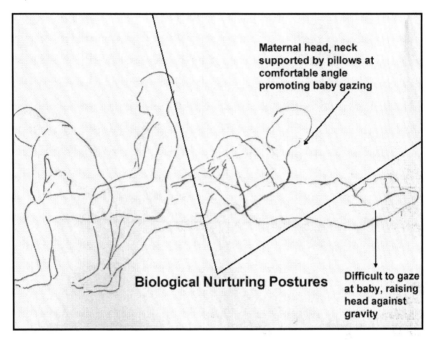

Figure 28. The Range of Biological Nurturing Postures
Line drawing © Suzanne Carter.

Having presented this theory at a recent National Childbirth Trust Conference, read below what one father, Mark Bendig, an English psychologist and Human Factors Consultant, wrote:

Hello Suzanne,

Here are some clarifications concerning our discussion about maternal flat-lying:

When mothers' hands are raised and above the body when supine, this naturally causes blood to drain from the fingers due to the effect of gravity. (Try lifting and holding your hands even a small distance above your shoulders and not only will you be able to feel the blood leave your hands more or less instantaneously, but you will quickly experience the sense of extreme fatigue that results when this is done for prolonged periods).

Although there are other complex factors involved, the end result is the loss of tactile sensitivity. For my work, this effect is very important when people must perform a critical task correctly whilst having to raise their hands and / or arms above the trunk, as doing so, even for short periods of time, results in extreme fatigue, which can take a long time to recover from (the effect is exacerbated by holding loads; the heavier they are, the more pronounced the effect is and the less time you can hold the load).

The interesting thing about new mums, it occurs to me, is that immediately following birth, blood pressure can be low (and may remain on the low side for sometime after birth). Recall it is blood pressure that determines how efficiently the heart can pump blood to and from the extremities: less pressure, less push.

The effect of this is to further reduce the heart's capability to pump blood to the fingertips with the hands raised. Add that mum will want to keep her hands raised, even if little effort is required to keep them up with baby, in order to hold and comfort baby, and it's not difficult to conceive that this posture is far from perfect for preserving sensitivity. Indeed, you may have noticed that when people are weak they cannot lift their hands? Of course, when the mother is flat-lying, the full weight of the baby will lie on mum's chest, this may also adversely affect heart function and hence impair circulation (try laying a heavy weight on your chest and see how much it affects respiration and heart rate!).

Given that you described at the conference women being flat on their backs and possibly having low blood pressure as a consequence of the birth event, it seems reasonable to postulate that there will be an increase in loss of tactile sensitivity. Another interesting thing is that it seems to me that mums might not attribute this weakness to posture; as they have been through a medical procedure; they could well be more inclined to attribute fatigue to other factors, such as exhaustion following birth or even the effect of drugs.

It seems to me that, given how important delicate tactile contact is for both mum and baby, anything that impairs sensitivity impairs any communication that may occur through this route from mum to baby and baby to mum.

As early as 1976, Klaus and Kennel described early maternal behaviours, citing a study carried out by Lang:

... the mother rubs the baby's skin, starting with the face. Rubbing is done with the fingertips and is usually a gentle stroking motion. This occurs before the initial nursing and before delivery of the placenta.
(Lang, 1972, p.69)

Taken together with Mark Bendig's observations, it can be suggested that a flat-lying maternal posture immediately following birth may reduce the impact of both the sensorial touching and gazing experiences, even when mothers and babies are in skin-to-skin contact.

Neonatal Prone and Flat-Lying: A Word of Caution

The individuality of maternal body slope, be it in skin-to-skin contact or when mothers and babies are lightly dressed, also accommodates the baby's need to be nursed in a physiological body tilt. When a mother lies perfectly flat on her back and places her baby on top, the baby lies prone and flat. This position, recognised since the early 1990s as suboptimal, places the neonate at risk of respiratory problems during the first postnatal months. Right after birth and during the first postnatal months, this is a position to be avoided, as the baby is making a cardiovascular transition. Nevertheless, we often see pictures of babies lying flat and prone during the first hour following birth to illustrate benefits of skin-to-skin contact (UNICEF India, 2007).

In contrast, a BN position where the baby is prone with a physiological body tilt head upward has proven developmental and respiratory benefits. For example, even though back to sleep is preferred, preterm infants are often nursed in prone positions, tilted upward to avoid reflux and to promote neonatal physiological stability in special care nurseries.

Hurst and Meier (2010, p. 436) state that "the position of the infant in STS [skin-to-skin] care is important in maintaining physiologic stability, and recliners are ideal in achieving this position... the recliner is angled back to allow the infant's body to remain at a 45 to 60 degree angle from the floor". This is a perfect biological nurturing position. Mothers do not need to purchase a recliner, but, of course, they can if they wish. It makes physiological sense to breastfeed and nurture any healthy baby (term, small for gestational age, and moderately preterm babies) in BN positions, in as much skin-to-skin contact as desired. The gentle body slope promotes neonatal locomotion and helps the newborn coordinate sucking and swallowing with breathing. Mothers will naturally adjust their degree of body slope to accommodate their individual baby's needs, as long as they are not advised to lie flat, placed in a flat-lying posture, or taught to sit upright.

Research Evidence

Before 2007, there were no randomised controlled trials examining skin-to-skin contact in laid-back maternal postures compared with babies lightly dressed in laid-back maternal postures. Bystrova and her colleagues (2007) looked at the effect of Russian maternity home routines on breastfeeding, with particular reference to swaddling and weight loss. There were six groups receiving a number of early and late manipulations comparing skin-to-skin contact, lightly dressed contact, and swaddling with dressed babies, in both separation and rooming-in situations.

For our purposes, the first two groups are of particular relevance: 37 babies were randomised to a skin-to-skin contact group and 40 to a lightly dressed contact group. The researchers specifically clarify the immediate postpartum maternal postures, as it seems that according to Russian practices at the time, all mothers were placed lying flat on their backs for the first two postnatal hours after birth. The randomised infants were returned to their mothers after a brief separation for about 20 minutes and placed prone on their mothers' bodies, either in skin-to-skin contact or lightly dressed, wearing identical sets of clothes, consisting of a cotton shirt with long sleeves, leggings, wool socks, and a cap.

Interestingly, when the researchers looked at outcomes on the fourth postnatal day, the results were similar for these two groups. There were no significant differences, although the lightly dressed group had a greater number of breastfeeds, lasting longer, and ingested, on average, more mother's milk than the skin-to-skin group; the only outcome for which the skin-to-skin group fared better concerned supplementation with artificial milk drink (5 mls for the skin-to-skin group compared to 8.7 mls for the lightly dressed group). Again, this difference was not significant.

Beyond the First Postnatal Hours

During the past ten years, there has been a real pressure put on parents to hold their babies in skin-to-skin contact, not just following birth, but whenever there is a breastfeeding problem. However, Bystrova et al. (2007) appear to replicate my research findings suggesting that being on the mother's body is the important factor. These observations, taken together with maternal reluctance to undress themselves or undress their babies, suggest that more research is needed before we suggest, for example, that "there are risks associated with not using skin-to-skin contact during the perinatal period" (Riordan & Hoover, 2010, p. 222).

Although repeatedly, randomised control trials (RCTs) have demonstrated thermal regulatory benefits, these studies have been carried out for the most part with the preterm population (Anderson et al., 2003). Term and preterm babies are completely different in their developmental needs and reactions. Yet few, if any, large RCTs using power calculations have examined thermal regulatory outcomes for healthy term infants. Nevertheless, proponents of early and prolonged skin-to-skin contact for healthy term infants claim that it:

- Increases breastfeeding duration.

- Results in less stress and greater maternal satisfaction with breastfeeding.

- Increases maternal desire to hold the baby.

- Mitigates the stress of being born and results in less crying (Riordan & Hoover, 2010).

All of these positive outcomes were also observed across the 40 mothers who tried BN, suggesting that we need to be cautious about extrapolating preterm results to the healthy term context, or assuming that all findings are due to skin-to-skin, rather than the mother's posture and the position of the baby.

Read below the testimonial received from a National Childbirth Trust (NCT) breastfeeding counsellor:

Dear Suzanne,

I am such a big fan of BN techniques and finding the whole idea just so refreshing and liberating for the mums I am in contact with, both antenatally and post. I did a breastfeeding antenatal session on Tuesday, and out of eight ladies, they all said without exception, that they felt so much more confident about establishing breastfeeding now that they had heard about BN (and having seen a little clip from the DVD). It would be great to get more midwives on board with it so that mums aren't left floundering during their time in hospital. :-)

Taken together, this evidence suggests that skin-to-skin contact and the positional impact need to be explored and discussed with mothers. Maybe some mothers do not want to share their naked frontal body region with their babies. Maybe a light amount of clothing can have protective effects. For example, Coles (2009) and Kendall-Tackett (2010) suggest that sexual assault survivors, in particular, may have difficulties with too much skin-to-skin contact. Being lightly dressed may make the contact more manageable.

These are some of the reasons that skin-to-skin contact is not listed as a constant variable of BN. Taken together these findings suggest that the jury is still out concerning the value of forcing mothers to breastfeed in skin-to-skin contact. At the same time, an increasing body of evidence supports the theoretical construct that feeding during the early weeks is primarily simple archaic reflex activity, reliant upon positional interactions. The 17 reconfigured PNRs are undoubtedly enhanced by heightened sensorial neonatal visual, olfactory, and tactile responses, but a naked frontal region, on the part of mother, baby, or both, is not an obligate component. In any case, breastfeeding in the biological nurturing context does not appear to consist of a group of learned (cognitive) skills associated with skin-to-skin contact during the time of initiation.

It is well known that the neocortex, covering the two hemispheres of the cerebrum, is responsible for cognition and intentionality. The neocortex is the least developed part of the brain at birth, suggesting that during the first postnatal hour, it is unlikely that neonatal interest, desire, or intention drives behaviours that initiate breastfeeding. It makes physiological sense that mammals be born with a number of innate, life-enhancing reflex movements to enable feeding; my study illustrates 20 such movements independent of variables such as early timing, a critical window, skin-to-skin contact, gestational age, and behavioural state.

BN is defined as a collective term for a range of breastfeeding positions where mothers are encouraged to hold their babies for as long and as often and in as much skin-to-skin contact as desired. Skin-to-skin contact is a mother's choice, not a biological imperative.

Chapter 12

Biological Nurturing: A Mother-Centred Approach

Mother-centeredness is a key aspect of BN. So often interest showered upon the mother during pregnancy can be perceived as foetal attention: the mother is the vessel carrying the baby (Rothman, 1985). As soon as the baby is born, some argue that all interest in the mother ends. Entire books are written about the amazing newborn. How many books do you know that are entitled the amazing mother? Observe how maternal-infant reciprocity unfolds in Figure 29.

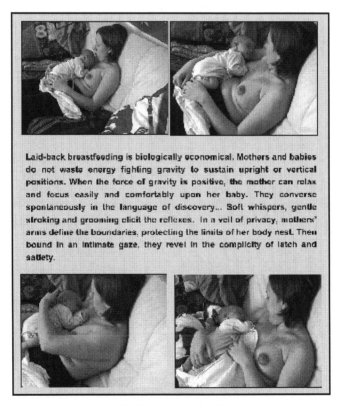

Figure 29. The Language of Discovery
Photos © Suzanne Colson.

My work suggests that mothers are truly amazing. Our research observations suggest that, in certain situations, whilst sacral sitting for example, mothers display spontaneous breastfeeding behaviours. Many mothers appeared to know instinctively how and when to release the reflexes.

In contrast, using current approaches to breastfeeding initiation, mothers often think they will fail at breastfeeding, even before they start! We use phrases like: "attempting or trying to breastfeed". When mothers ask questions, instead of sharing our confidence in the unique biological design of a mother's body to nourish and nurture her baby, health professionals often suggest metaphors, saying that breastfeeding is like typing, riding a bike, dancing, or driving a car. These metaphors are not entirely accurate. These types of activities are learned skills and/or enhancements to increase enjoyment of life or to get ahead professionally, but they are neither necessary to sustain life nor integral to a life-long relationship.

Nursing your baby lays the foundations for a life-long relationship. Breastfeeding is comparable to those activities of daily living as defined in the Roper, Logan, and Tierney (2000) model of nursing. Breastfeeding, in itself, maintains a safe environment and is an activity that is associated with breathing, communication, personal hygiene, mobility, eating, drinking, and expressing sexuality among others. The suggestion that breastfeeding is similar to learned activities often creates a "helpless" mother, dependent upon advice from experts at the very time when new-mothers feel most vulnerable.

Biologically, and in countries untouched by lactation management, breastfeeding remains an activity of daily living for an average of four years for both mother and baby. There is mutual dependency when it is supposed to happen, at just the right time in the life span. Breastfeeding is certainly not something that the baby does by himself as some have suggested.

The word relationship implies, by definition, the give and take of two people. Mothers are active breastfeeders! They guide and protect their babies, aiding latch as necessary through what we have observed as "emerging sequential patterns of maternal instinctual behaviours" (Colson et al., 2008, p. 446). Furthermore, mothers' participation is essential; human mothers do not lie inert, rather they elicit reciprocal innate behavioural patterns creating mother-child ties based upon love and respect. Mothers know more about their babies than anyone. They constantly assess their babies' well-being, detecting as soon as possible any deviation from normal or potential problems.

The breastfeeding relationship, like any relationship, comprises both innate and acquired behaviours. However, for over a century, the *breastfeeding as an acquired skill*–or the nurturing approach–has dominated our understanding and informed practice about how mothers best initiate breastfeeding. Biological Nurturing restores balance, bringing the nature or innate component back into breastfeeding.

Innate reproductive behaviours depend upon the right hormonal environment. The BN approach emphasises, first and foremost, the importance of maintaining an environment conducive to the release of the primary breastfeeding hormones, oxytocin and prolactin. It promotes mothers' self-discovery and then observes maternal behaviours, learning from mothers and trusting maternal instincts to release baby behaviours.

References

Als, H. (1995). Manual for the naturalistic observation of newborn behavior. *Newborn Individualized Developmental Care and Assessment Program* (NIDCAP). Boston: The Children's Hospital.

Amiel-Tison, C., & Grenier, A. (1984). *La Surveillance Neurologique au cours de la Première Année de la Vie.* Paris: Masson.

Anderson, G.C. (1989). Skin-to-skin: Kangaroo care in Western Europe. *American Journal of Nursing, 89,* 662-666.

Anderson, G.C., Moore, E., Hepworth, J., & Bergman, N. (2003). Early skin-to-skin contact for mothers and their healthy newborn infants. *The Cochrane Database of Systematic Reviews,* Issue 2.

Anderson, G.C., Chiu, S.H., Morrison, B., Burkhammer, M., & Ludington-Hoe, S. (2004). Skin-to-skin care for breastfeeding difficulties postbirth. In T. Field (Ed.), *Touch and massage in early child development.* Miami, FL: Johnson & Johnson Pediatric Institute.

André-Thomas, J.M., Chesni, Y., & Saint-Anne Dargassies, S. (1960). *The neurological examination of the infant.* The Medical Advisory Committee of the National Spastic Society: London.

Balaskas, J. (1983). *Active birth.* London: Unwin Paperbacks.

Bentley, G.R. (1998). Hydration as a limiting factor in lactation. *American Journal of Human Biology. 10,* 151-161.

Bergman, N. (2010). Restoring the original paradigm for infant care. *Kangaroo Mother Care Promotions.* Retrieved on 24 May 2010, from http://www.kangaroomothercare.com/prevtalk01.htm.

Biancuzzo, M. (1999). *Breastfeeding the newborn. Clinical strategies for nurses.* St Louis: Mosby.

Blackburn, S.T. (2003). *Maternal, fetal, and neonatal physiology: A clinical perspective* (2nd ed.). St Louis, MO: W.B. Saunders Company.

Bolling K., Grant, C., Hamlyn, B., & Thornton, K. (2007). *Infant feeding survey 2005.* London: The Information Centre.

Bragg, M. (1991). [abstract and review] Righard L. & Alade, M.O. (1990). Effect of delivery room routines on success of first breast-feed. Lancet, 336, 8723, 1105-1107 in MIDIRS Midwifery Digest Review No. 901031 Standard Search L46, PN101. Retrieved 20 March 2006 from http://www.MIDIRS.org or on Ovid: Maternity and Infant Care Data Base (accessed 16 June 2010).

Brazelton, T.B. (1973). Effect of maternal expectations on early infant behaviour. *Early Child Development and Care, 2,* 259 –273.

Brazelton, T.B., & Nugent, J.K. (1995). *Neonatal behavioral assessment scale* (3rd ed.). London: Mac Keith Press.

Brazelton, T.B., & Nugent, J.K. (1999). *Neonatal behavioral assessment scale* [videocassette]. Boston: The Brazelton Institute Children's Hospital Boston, Harvard Medical School.

Brown, L. (1993). *The new shorter Oxford dictionary* (5th ed.). Oxford: Oxford University Press.

Brown, M.S., & Hurlock, J. T. (1975). Preparation of the breast for breastfeeding. *Nursing Research, 24*(6), 448-451.

Bullough, C.H.W., Msuku, R.S., & Karonde, L. (1989). Early suckling and postpartum haemorrhage: Controlled trial in deliveries by traditional birth attendants. *The Lancet, 9,* 522-525.

Bystrova, K., Matthiesen A.S., Widstrom, A.M., Ransjo-Arvidson, A.B., Welles-Nystrom, B., Vorontsov, I., et al. (2007). The effect of Russian maternity home routines on breastfeeding and neonatal weight loss with special reference to swaddling. *Early Human Development, 83,* 29-39.

Cadogan, W. (1748). *An essay upon nursing, and the management of children: From their birth to three years of age.* London: Published by Order of the General Committee for transacting the Affairs of the Foundling Hopsital. Reprinted for J. Roberts in Warwick-Lane.

Christensson, K., Siles, C., Moreno, A. Belaustequi, A., de La Fuente, P., Lagercrantz, H., et al. (1992). Temperature, metabolic adaptation and crying in healthy full-term newborns cared for skin-to-skin or in a cot. *Acta Paediatrica, 81,* 488-493.

Christensson, K., Cabrera, T., Christensson, E., Uvnäs-Moberg, K., & Winberg, J. (1995). Separation and distress call in the human neonate in the absence of maternal body contact. *Acta Paediatrica, 84,* 466-473.

Cockburn, K. G., & Drake, R.F. (1969). Transverse and oblique lie of the foetus. *Obstetrical & Gynecological Survey, 24*(10), 1253-1255.

Coles, J. (2009). Qualitative study of breastfeeding after childhood sexual assault. *Journal of Human Lactation, 25*(3), 317-324.

Colson, S. (1997a). From conception to birth and beyond. *Midwives, 110,* 1309, 40-41.

Colson, S. (1997b). A baby feeding advisor: Who needs one? *Midwifery Matters, 72,* 14-17.

Colson, S. (2000). *Biological suckling facilitates exclusive breastfeeding from birth a pilot study of twelve vulnerable infants.* Unpublished master's dissertation. London: South Bank University.

Colson, S. (2002). Womb to world: A metabolic perspective. *Midwifery Today. 46* (1), 12-17.

Colson, S. (2005a). Maternal breastfeeding positions, have we got it right? (1). *The Practising Midwife, 8,* 10, 24-27.

Colson, S. (2005b). Maternal breastfeeding positions, have we got it right? (2). *The Practising Midwife, 8,* 11, 29-32.

Colson, S. (2007). Biological nurturing (2) the physiology of lactation revisited. *The Practising Midwife, 10* (10), 14-19.

Colson, S. (2008). Bringing nature to the fore. *Practising Midwife, 11* (10), 14-16,18-19.

Colson, S., DeRooy, L., & Hawdon, J. (2003). Biological nurturing increases breastfeeding duration. *MIDIRS Midwifery Digest, 13* (1), 92-97.

Colson, S., Frantz, K., & Makelin, I. (2010). *Biological Nurturing for Mothers* [DVD]. Geddes Productions. Available online at http://www.geddesproduction.com/.

Colson, S., & Greenfield, T. (2006). Maternal hormonal complexion, a theory. In S. Colson, *The mechanisms of biological nurturing.* Doctoral thesis, Canterbury Christ Church University, Canterbury, UK.

Colson, S., & Giffiths, H. (1996). Breastfeeding: Rediscovery of the lost art. *Nursing Times, 92,* 11, 59-64.

Colson, S.D., Meek J.H., & Hawdon, J.M. (2008). Optimal positions for the release of primitive neonatal reflexes stimulating breastfeeding. *Early Human Development, 84,* 441-449. Available online at http://linkinghub.elsevier.com/retrieve/pii/S0378378207002423.

Darwin, C. (1872). Biographical sketch of a small child. In A. Peiper. (1963). *Cerebral Function in Infancy and Childhood* (B. Nagler & H. Nagler, Trans.). New York: Consultants Bureau, 417.

De Château, P., & Wiberg, B. (1977). Long-term effect on mother-infant behavior of extra contact during the first hour postpartum. I. First observations at 36 hours. *Acta Paediatrica Scandinavica, 66,* 137-143.

De Château, P. (1987). Left-sided preference in holding and carrying newborn infants: A three-year follow-up study. *Acta Psychiatrica Scandinavica, 75,* 283-286.

De Gasquet, B. (2005). *Bébé est la, vive maman, les suites de couches.* Paris: Robert Jauze.

De Rooy, L., & Hawdon, J.M. (2002). Nutritional factors that affect the postnatal metabolic adaptation of full-term small and large for gestational age infants. *Pediatrics, 109,* 42. Retrieved on 24 May 2010 from http://pediatrics.aappublications.org/cgi/content/full/109/3/e42.

Dick-Read, G. (1954). *Childbirth without fear.* New York: Harper and Row.

Dubowitz, L., Dubowitz, V., & Mercuri E. (1999). The neurological assessment of the preterm and the full term newborn infant. Clinics in developmental medicine. *Spastics International Medical Publications.* Philadelphia: JB Lippincott, No. 79.

Elman, J.L., Bates, E.A., Johnson, M.H., Karmiloff-Smith, A., Parisi, D., & Plunkett, K. (1998). *Rethinking innateness: A connectionist perspective on development.* Michigan: MIT Press Paperback.

Foster K., Lader, D., & Cheesbrough S. (1997). *Infant feeding 1995.* Office for National Statistics. London: The Stationery Office.

Gaskin, I.M. (1977). *Spiritual midwifery.* Summertown, TN: The Book Publishing Company.

Gesell, A., Ilg, F.L., & Ames, L.B. (1974). *Infant and child in the culture of today.* London: Hamish Hamilton.

Gohil, J.R. (2006). Boxing neonate on an engorged breast: A new behavior identified. *Journal of Human Lactation, 23,* 3, 268–269.

Gunther, M. (1955). Instinct & the nursing couple. *Lancet, 265,* 6864, 575-578.

Hamlyn, B., Brooker, S., Oleinikova, K., & Wands S. (2002). *Infant feeding 2000.* London: TSO.

Hardyment, C. (1983). *Dream babies child care from Locke to Spock.* London: Jonathan Cape.

Hartmann, P.E., & Prosser, C.G. (1984). Physiological basis of longitudinal changes in human milk yield and composition. *Federation Proceedings, 43,* 2448-2453.

Hartmann, P.E. (1987). Lactation and reproduction in Western Australian women. *Reproductive Medicine, 32,* 543-547.

Hawdon, J.M., Ward Platt, M.P., & Aynsley-Green, A. (1992). Patterns of metabolic adaptation in term and preterm infants in the first postnatal week. *Archives of Diseases of Childhood, 67,* 357-365.

Hawdon, J.M., Ward Platt, M.P., & Aynsley-Green, A. (1993). Neonatal hypoglycaemia/ blood glucose monitoring and baby feeding. *Midwifery, 9,* 3-6.

Henderson, C., & MacDonald, S. (2004). *Mayes' midwifery* (13th ed.). London: Balliere Tindall.

Herbert, J. (1994). Oxytocin and sexual behaviour. *British Medical Journal, 309,* 891-892.

Hoseth, E., Joergensen, A., Ebbesen, F., & Moeller, M. (2000). Blood glucose levels in a population of healthy breastfed term infants of appropriate size for gestational age. *Archives of Diseases of Childhood. Fetal Neonatal Edition, 83,* F117-F119.

Howie, P.W. (1985). Breastfeeding: A new understanding. *Midwives Chronicle and Nursing Notes, 7,* 184-192.

Howie, P.W., Houston, M.J., Cook, A., Smart, L., McArdle, T., & McNeilly, A.S. (1981). How long should a breast-feed last? *Early Human Development, 5,* 71-77.

Hurst, N.M., & Meier, P.P. (2010). Breastfeeding the preterm infant. In J. Riordan & K. Wambach (Eds.), *Breastfeeding and human lactation* (4th ed.). Boston, MA: Jones & Bartlett.

Hytten, F. (1995). *The clinical physiology of the puerperium.* London: Perrand Press.

Illingworth, R.S. (1963). *The development of the infant and young child: Normal and abnormal* (2nd ed.). Edinburgh: E. & S. Livingstone Ltd.

Inch, S. (2003). Confusion surrounding breastfeeding terms 'positioning' and 'attachment'. *BJM (letter), 11,* 3, 148.

Kapandji, I.A. (1974). *The physiology of the joints*. Vol.3. *The trunk and the vertebral column* (2nd ed.). Edinburgh: Churchill Livingstone.

Kendall-Tackett, K. (2010). *Depression in new mothers: Causes, consequences, and treatment alternatives* (2nd ed.). London: Routledge.

Kitzinger, S. (1972). *The experience of childbirth* (3rd ed.). Middlesex, UK: Penguin.

Klaus, M.H., & Kennel, J.H. (1976). *Maternal-infant bonding* (1st American ed.). St Louis, MO: Mosby Company.

Klaus, M.H., & Klaus, P.H. (1985). *The amazing newborn.* Reading, MA: Addison-Wesley Publishing Company Inc.

Koehn, M., & Riordan, J. (2010). Infant assessment. In J. Riordan & K. Wambach (Eds.), *Breastfeeding and human lactation* (4th ed.). Boston, MA: Jones & Bartlett.

Lang, R. (1972). *Birth book.* Ben Lomond, CA: Genesis Press.

Leboyer, F. (1974). *Pour une naissance sans violence.* Paris: Editions Le Seuil.

Lorenz, K. (1952). *King Solomon's ring.* London: Methuen & Co Ltd.

Ludington-Hoe, S.M., with Golant, S.K. (1993). *Kangaroo care.* New York: Bantam Books.

Martin, J., & Monk, J. (1982). *Infant feeding 1980.* Office of Population Censuses and Surveys. London: Social Survey Division, HMSO.

Martin, J., & White, A. (1987). *Infant feeding 1985.* Office of population Censuses and Surveys. London: Social Survey Division, HMSO.

Matthiesen, A.S., Ransjo-Arvidson, A.B., Nissen, E., & Uvnäs-Mobert, K. (2001). Postpartum maternal oxytocin release by newborns: Effects of infant hand massage and sucking. *Birth, 28*(1), 13-19.

McFarland, D. (2006). *A dictionary of animal behaviour.* Oxford, UK: Oxford University Press.

McNabb, M. (1997a). Maternal and fetal physiological responses to pregnancy. In B.R. Sweet, with D. Tiran (Eds.), *Mayes' midwifery* (12th ed.). London: Balliere Tindall.

McNabb, M. (1997b). The physiology of lactation. In B.R. Sweet, with D. Tiran, (Eds.). *Mayes' midwifery* (12th ed.). London: Balliere Tindall.

McNabb, M., & Colson, S. (2000). From pregnancy to lactation: Changing relations between mother and baby/a biological perspective. In J. Alexander, C. Roth, & V. Levy (Eds.). *Midwifery practice core topics, 3,* 51-65.

McNeilly, A.S., Robinson, I.C.A., Houston, M.J., & Howie, P.W. (1983). Release of oxytocin and prolactin in response to suckling. *British Medical Journal, 286,* 257-259.

Medical Research Council (MRC). (2000). *Framework for the development and evaluation of complex interventions.* Retrieved 10 February 2003 from http://www.mrc.ac.uk.

Montagu, A. (1965). *Life before birth.* New York: Signet.

Montagu, A. (1971). *Touching: The human significance of the skin.* New York: Harper & Row Publishers.

Moore, E.R., & Anderson, G.C. (2005). Randomized controlled trial or early mother-infant skin-to-skin contact and breastfeeding success. *Journal of Human Lactation, 21*(4), 488–489.

Morris, D. (1977). *Manwatching :A field guide to human behaviour.* London: Triad/Panther Ltd.

National Childbirth Trust. (1997). Hypoglycaemia of the newborn: New guidelines now available. *New Generation Digest, 19,* 9. London: National Childbirth Trust.

Nijhuis, J.G., Prechtl, H.F.R., Martin Jr. C. B., & Botts, R.S.G.M. (1982). Are there behavioural states in the human fetus? *Early Human Development, 6*(2), 177-195.

Nissen, E., Uvnäs-Moberg, K., Svensson, K., Stock, S., Widstrom, A.M., & Winberg, J. (1996). Different patterns of oxytocin, prolactin but not cortisol release during breastfeeding in women delivered by Caesarean section or by the vaginal route. *Early Human Development, 45,* 103-118.

Nyqvist, K.H. (2005). Breastfeeding support in neonatal care: An example of the integration of international evidence and experience. *Newborn and Infant Nursing Reviews, 5*(1), 34–48.

Odent, M. (1977). The early expression of the rooting reflex. *Proceedings of the 5th international congress of psychosomatics, obstetrics and gynaecology, Rome* (pp. 1117-1119). London: Academic Press.

Odent, M. (1984). *Birth reborn.* London: Souvenir Press.

Odent, M. (1987). The fetus ejection reflex. *Birth, 14,* 104-105.

Odent, M. (1992). *The nature of birth and breastfeeding.* Westport, CT: Bergin and Garvey.

Odent, M. (1999). *The scientification of love.* London: Free Association Books.

Odent, M. (2002). The first hour following birth: Don't wake the mother. *Midwifery Today, 61,* 9-11.

Odent, M. (2004). *The caesarean.* London: Free Association Books.

Pedersen, C.A. (1992). Oxytocin in maternal sexual and social behaviours. *Annals of the New York Academy of Sciences, 652,* IX-XI.

Peiper, A.(1963). *Cerebral function in infancy and childhood* (3rd ed.) (B. Nagler & H. Nagler, Trans.). New York: Consultants Bureau.

Piaget, J. (1955). *The child's construction of reality*. London: Routledge and Kegan Paul Ltd.

Prechtl, H. & Schleidt, W.M. (1951). In Peiper, A. (1963). *Cerebral Function in Infancy and Childhood* (B. Nalger & H. Nagler, Trans.). New York: Consultants Bureau, 161.

Prechtl, H.F.R. (1974). The behavioural states of the newborn infant (A Review). *Brain Research, 76,* 185-212.

Prechtl, H. (1977). *The neurological examination of the full term new born infant* (2nd ed.). Clinics in Developmental Medicine, No 63. London: William Heinemann Books Ltd (Spastic International Medical Publications).

Prechtl, H. (2001). General movement assessment as a method of developmental neurology: New paradigms and their consequences: The Ronnie MacKeith Lecture 1999. *Developmental Medicine and Child Neurology, 43,* 12, 836-842.

Preyer, W. (1893). *The mind of a child, part I: The senses and the will* (pp. 1-17). New York: Appleton. In J. F. Rosenblith and J. E. Sims-Knight. (1985). *In the beginning: Development in the first two years*. Monterey CA: Brooks/Cole. Publishing Company.

Pryor, K. (1963). *Nursing your baby* (1st ed.). New York: Harper & Row.

Quandt, S.A. (1998). Ecology of breastfeeding in the United States: An applied perspective. *American Journal of Human Biology, 10,* 221-228.

Reader, F. (1996). The hospital experience. In K. Moss (Ed.). *Hidden loss* (2nd ed.). London: The Women's Press.

Renfrew, M., Woolridge, M.W., & McGill, H.R. (2000). *Enabling breastfeeding*. London: TSO.

Renfrew, M., Dyson, L., Wallace, L., D'Souza, L., McCormick, F., & Spiby, H. (2005). *The effectiveness of public health interventions to promote the duration of breastfeeding systematic review* (1st ed.). London: National Institute for Health and Clinical Excellence (NICE).

Rey, E.S., & Martinez, H.G. (1983). *Manejo rational de nino prematuro*. Proceedings of the conferences held at Bogota, Colombia, March 17-19, 1983 [Spanish]: 137-151.

Righard, L., & Alade, M.O. (1990). Effects of delivery room routines on success of first feed. *The Lancet, 336,* 1105-1107.

Righard, L., & Frantz, K. (1992). *Delivery self attachment* [videocassette]. Sunland, CA: Geddes Productions.

Righard, L. (1995). How do newborns find their mother's breast? *Birth, 22,* 3, 174-175.

Riordan, J., & Hoover, K. (2010). Perinatal and intrapartum care. In J. Riordan & K. Wambach (Eds.), *Breastfeeding and human lactation* (4th ed.). Boston, MA: Jones & Bartlett.

Roper, N., Logan, W.W., & Tierney, A.J. (2000). *The Roper, Logan, and Tierney model of nursing based on activities of living* (4th ed.). London: Churchill Livingstone.

Rothman, B.K. (1985). *In Labour: Women and power in the birthplace*. London: Junction books Ltd.

Slater, A., Hocking, I., & Loose, J. (2003). Theories and issues in child development. In A. Slater & G. Bremner (Eds.). *An introduction to developmental psychology* (pp. 34-64). Oxford: Blackwell Publishing.

Sulcova, E. (1997). *Prague newborn behaviour description technique: manual.* Prague: Psychiatric Center, Laboratory of Psychometric Studies.

Tew, M. (1995). *Safer Childbirth: A critical history of maternity care* (2nd ed.). London: Chapman & Hall.

Thompson, D. (1995). *The Concise Oxford Dictionary* (9th Edition). Oxford: Clarendon Press.

Thureen, P.J., Deacon, J., Hernandez, J. & Hall, D. (2004). *Assessment and care of the well newborn.* Philadelphia: W.B. Saunders Company.

Tinbergen, N. (1951). *The study of instinct.* Oxford: Clarendon Press.

Truby King, F.T. (1924). *The expectant mother, and baby's first months.* London: Macmillan.

Truby King, M. (1934) *Mothercraft.* London: Simpkin, Marshall Ltd.

UNICEF. (2010). The Baby Friendly Initiative. Retrieved 7 May, 2010, from http://www.babyfriendly.org.uk.

UNICEF India. (2007). *Breast crawl: Initiation of breastfeeding by breast crawl* [videocassette]. Mumbai India: UNICEF Maharashtra. Retrieved on 10 May 2010 from http://breastcrawl.org/.

Uvnäs-Moberg, K. (1989). Physiological and psychological effects of oxytocin and prolactin in connection with motherhood with special reference to food intake and the endocrine system of the gut. *Acta Physiologica Scandinavica, 136 Supplementum, 583,* 41-48.

Uvnäs-Moberg, K. (1996). Neuroendocrinology of the mother-child interaction. *Trends in Endocrinology and Metabolism, 7 (*4), 126-131.

Uvnäs-Moberg, K. (1997). Oxytocin linked antistress effects–the relaxation and growth response. *Acta Physiologica Scandinavia Supplementum, 584,* 38-42.

Uvnäs-Moberg, K. (1998). Antistress pattern induced by oxytocin. *News in Physiological Science, 13,* 22-26.

Uvnäs-Moberg, K. (2003). *The oxytocin factor.* Cambridge, MA: Da Capo Press.

Wagner, M. (2006). *Born in the USA: How a broken maternity system must be fixed to put mothers and infants first.* Berkeley, CA: University of California Press.

Varendi, H., Porter, R.H., & Winberg, J. (1994). Does the newborn baby find the nipple by smell? *The Lancet, 344,* 989-990.

Walker, M. (Ed.). (2002). *International Lactation Consultant's Association: Core curriculum for lactation consultant practice.* Sudbury, MA: Jones and Bartlett Publishers.

White, A., Freeth, S., & O'Brien, M. (1992). *Infant feeding 1990.* London: OPCS Social Survey Division HMSO.

Widstrom, A.M., Ransjo-Arvidson, A.B., Matthiesen, A.S., Winberg, J., & Uvnäs-Moberg, K. (1987). Gastric suction in healthy newborn infants. *Acta Paediatrica Scandanavica, 76,* 566-572.

Widstrom, A.M. (1996). *Breastfeeding: Baby's choice* [Videocassette]. Stockholm: Liber Utbildning. Winberg, J. (1995). Examining breast feeding performance: Forgotten influencing factors. *Acta Paediatrica, 84,* 465-467.

Wolff, P.H. (1959). Observations on newborn Infants. *Psychosomatic Medicine, 21,* 110-118.

Wolff, P.H. (1966). The causes, controls and organisation of behaviour in the neonate. *Psychological Issues Monograph Series,* Vol. 5(1). New York: International Universities Press.

Wolff, P.H. (1987). *The development of behavioral states and the expression of emotion in early infancy.* Chicago: The University of Chicago Press.

Wood, E.C., & Forster, F.M. (2005). Oblique and transverse foetal lie. *Obstetric and Gynecological Clinics of North America, 32 (2),* 165-179.

Woolridge, M.W. (1986a). The 'anatomy' of infant sucking. *Midwifery, 2,* 164-171.

Woolridge, M.W. (1986b). Aetiology of sore nipples. *Midwifery, 2,* 172-176.

World Health Organization (WHO). (1997). *Breast-feeding management: A modular course.* London: WHO/UNICEF.

World Health Organization (WHO). (1998). *Evidence for the ten steps to successful breastfeeding* (Revised). Family and Reproductive Health Division of Child Health and Development. Geneva: World Health Organization.

Index

Author Bio

Suzanne Colson is an independent midwifery lecturer and an honorary senior lecturer at Canterbury Christ Church University. She has 35 years experience supporting breastfeeding mothers in both hospital and community settings. She is a Royal College of Nursing Akinsanya Scholar 2007, an honorary member and founding mother/leader of La Leche League France, and a member of the LLL professional advisory panel in the UK and France. Dr. Colson is the author of the DVD, *Biological Nurturing ~ Laid-Back Breastfeeding* for health professionals. A new DVD for parents will be available through Geddes Productions in September 2010. She has also written research papers, articles, and information sheets, some of which are available on the biological nurturing web site www.biologicalnurturing.com.

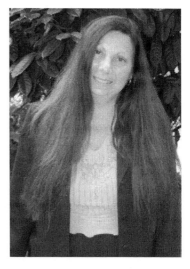

Dr. Colson worked in France as a lactation consultant with Michel Odent, and as a caseload midwife to French-speaking asylum seekers in London and a midwife/baby feeding advisor in London hospitals. Passionate about research, she worked on the Williams, Hawdon, and DeRooy team, examining the effects of supplementation on metabolic adaptation and breastfeeding and studied a subset of mother/baby pairs for her MSc. She was awarded a doctorate in 2006 for her work examining the mechanisms of biological nurturing; the thesis won first prize in the inaugural Akinsanya contest, a prestigious award given by the Royal College of Nursing Research Society for originality and scholarship in doctoral studies.

62345598R00076

Made in the USA
Charleston, SC
14 October 2016